# Visions of Cardiomyocyte - Fundamental Concepts of Heart Life and Disease

*Edited by Angelos Tsipis*

Published in London, United Kingdom

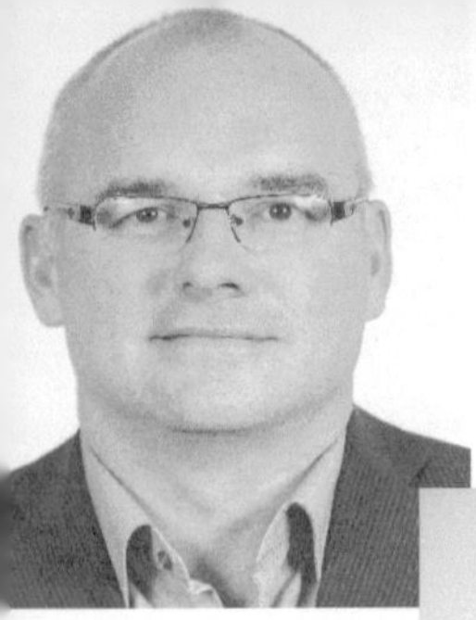
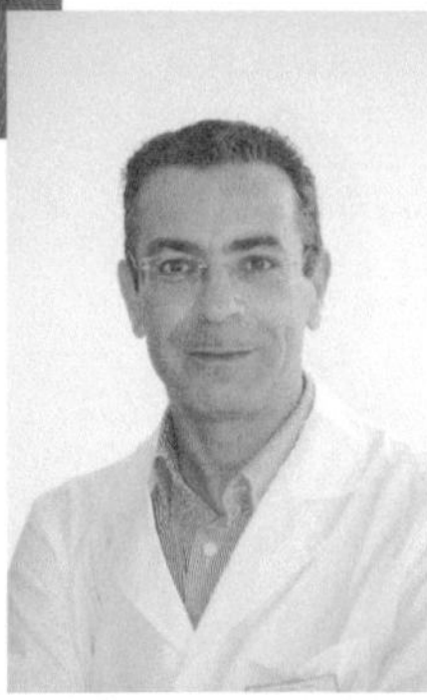
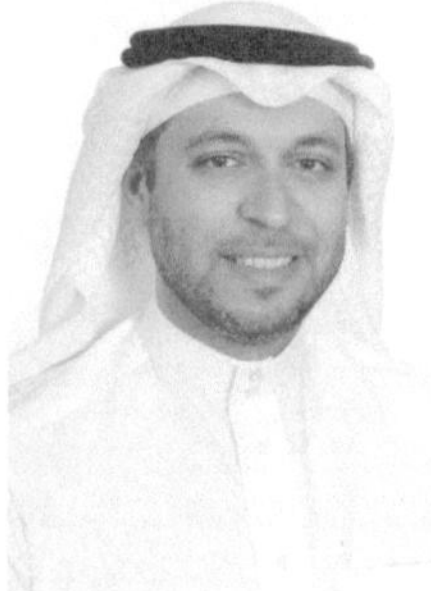
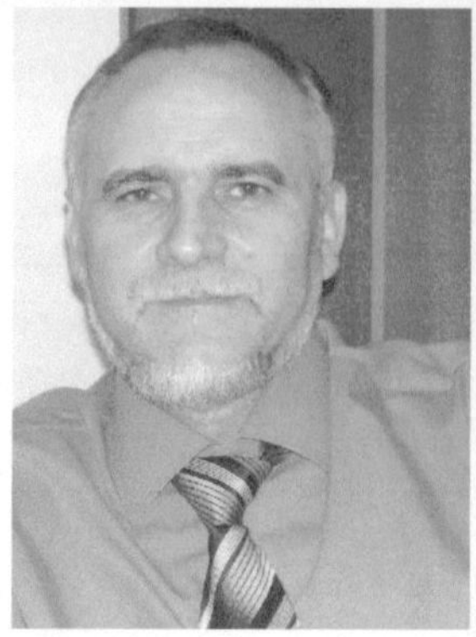
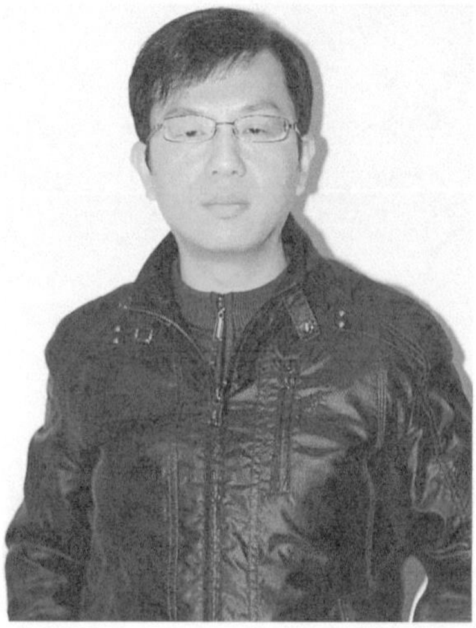
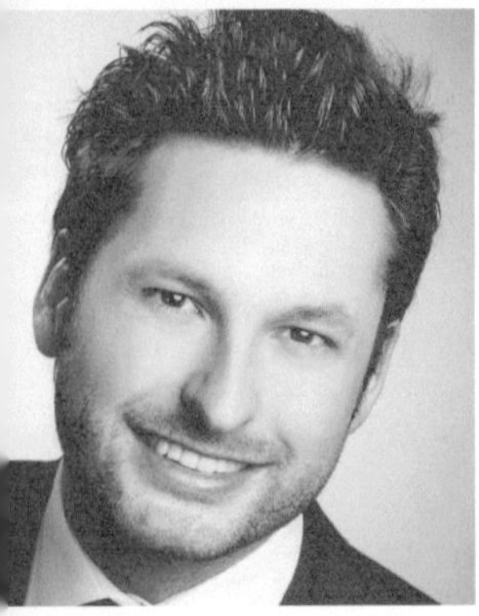
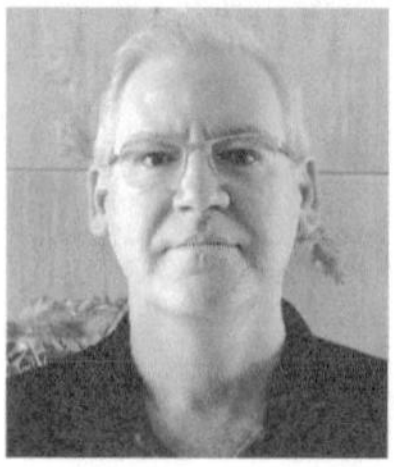

IntechOpen

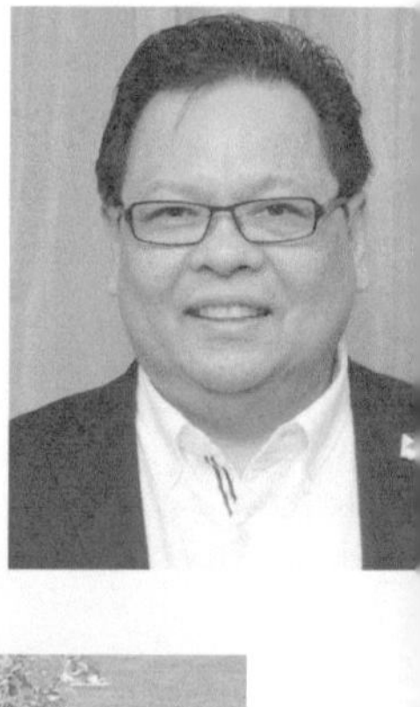
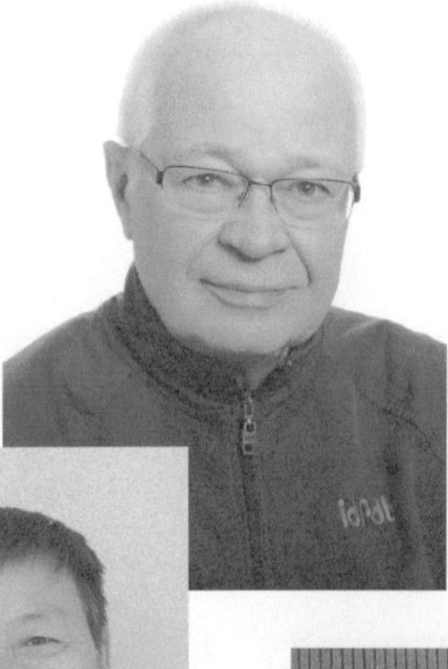
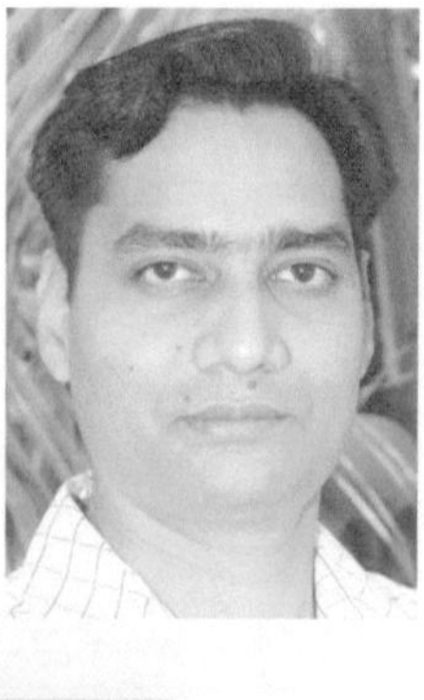
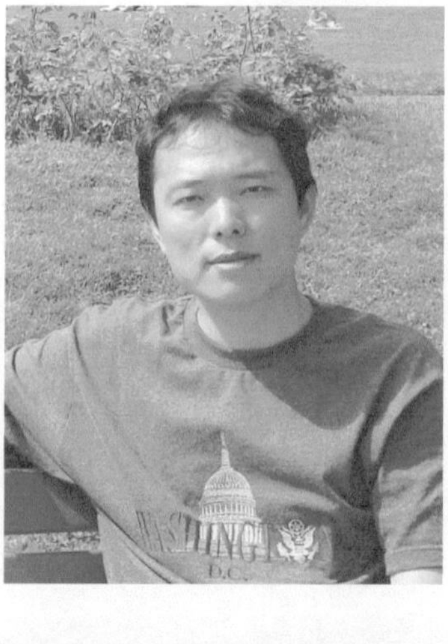
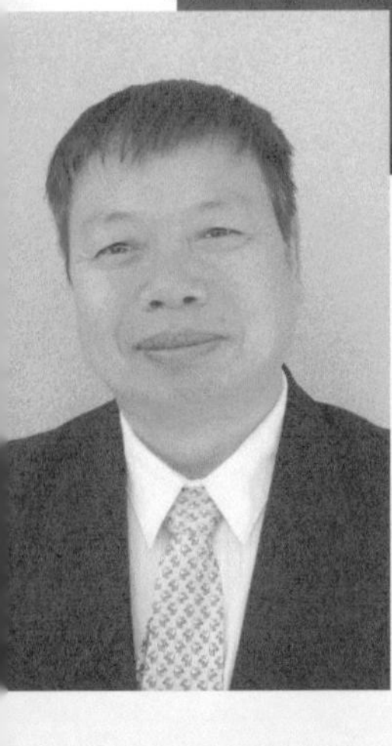
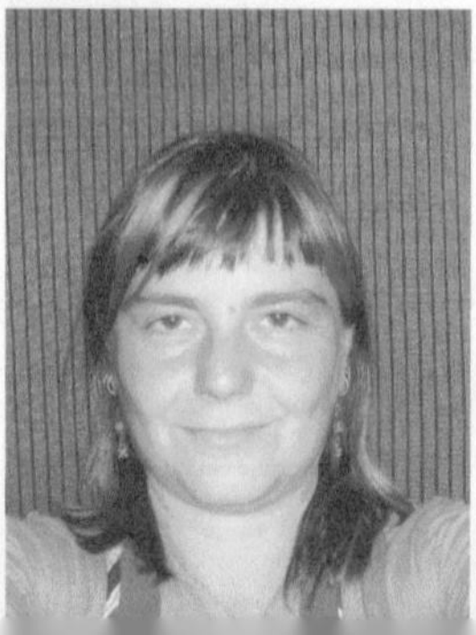

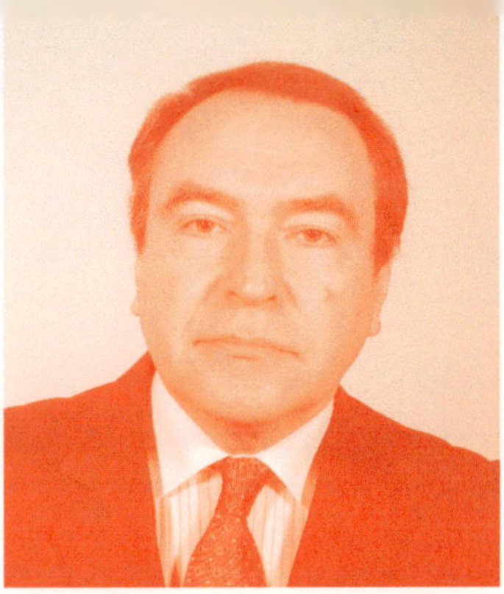
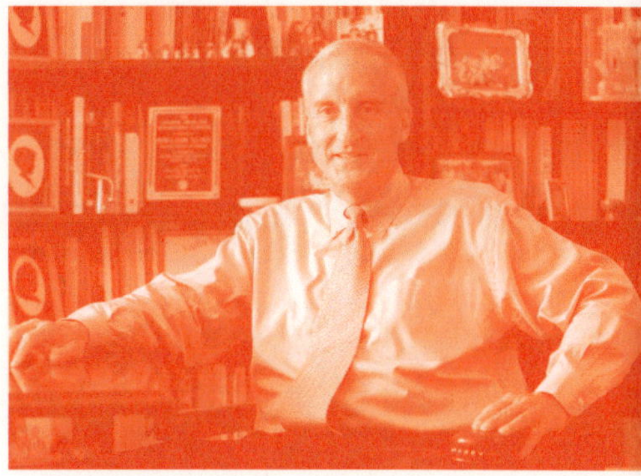
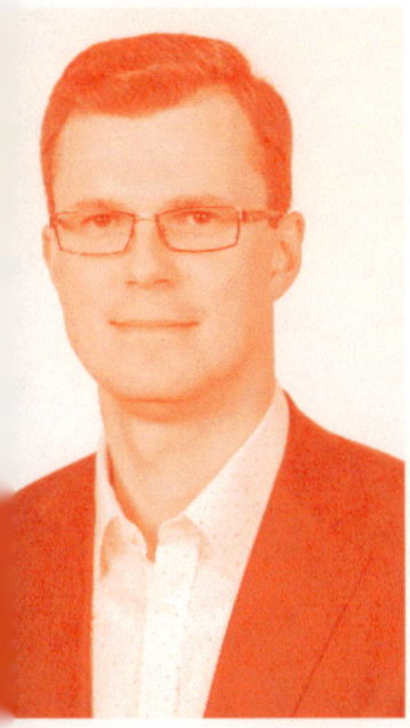
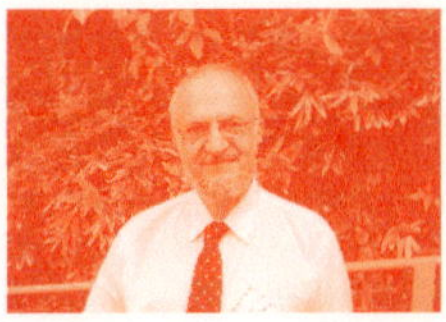
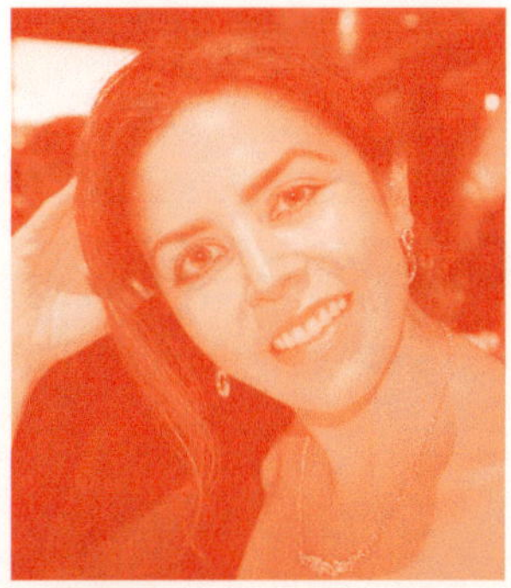

*Supporting open minds since 2005*

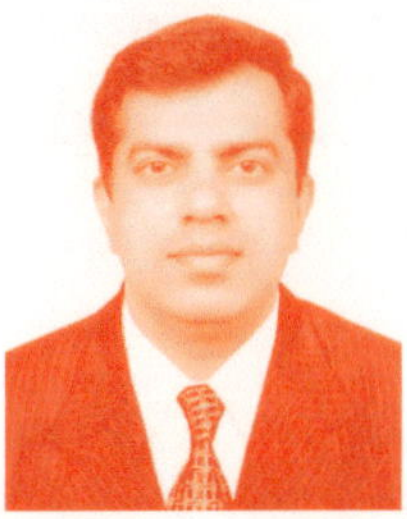
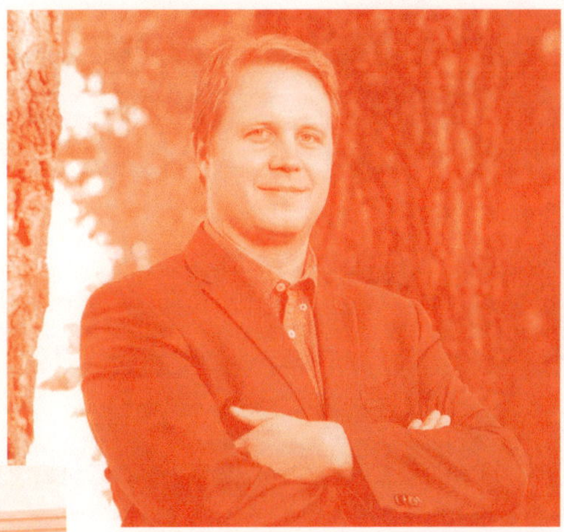
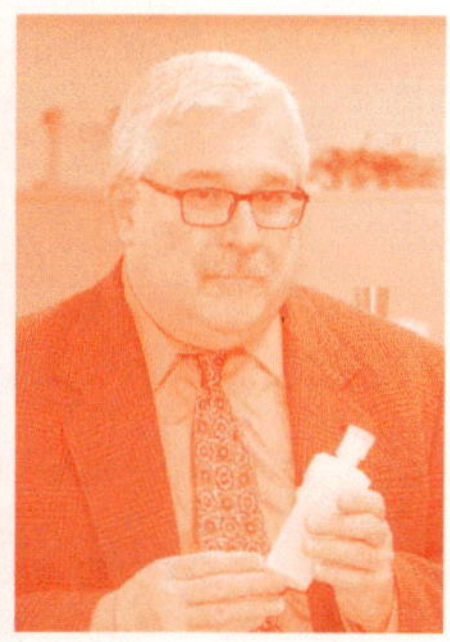
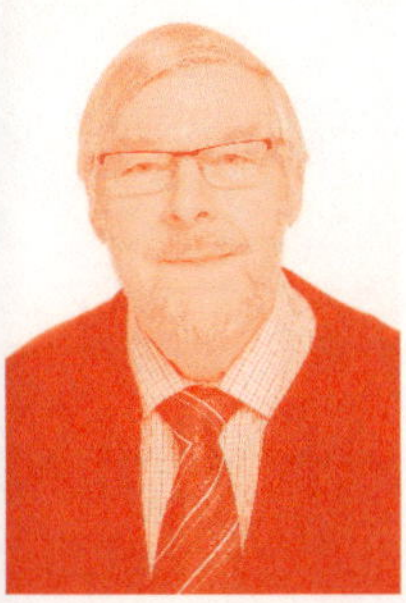
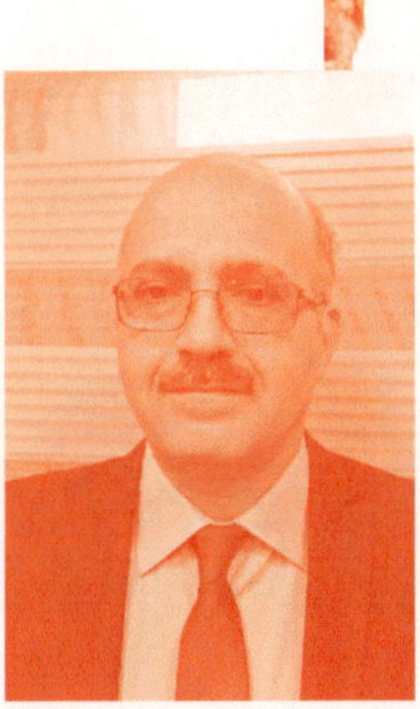
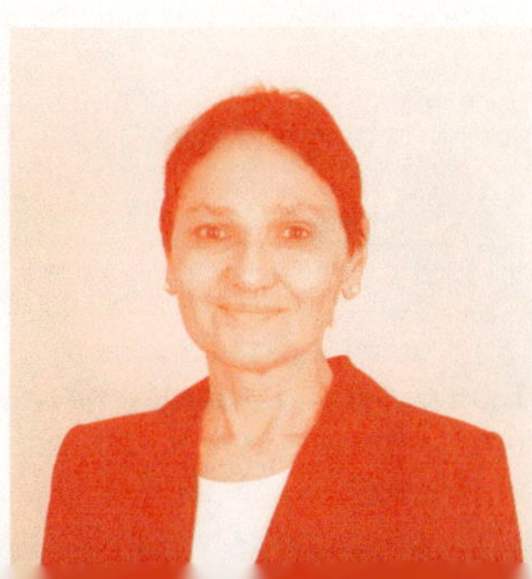
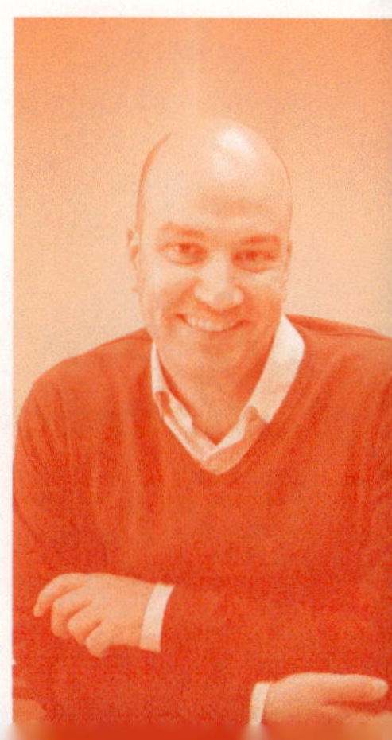

Visions of Cardiomyocyte - Fundamental Concepts of Heart Life and Disease
http://dx.doi.org/10.5772/intechopen.79311
Edited by Angelos Tsipis

Contributors
Ivana Škrlec, Svjetlana Marić, Aleksandar Včev, Marco Antonio Lopez Hernandez, Klaus-Dieter Schlüter, Rolf Schreckenberg, Nisha Arenja, Deborah P. Schild, Sascha I. Ricciardi, Jens G. Hellige, Rolf Vogel, Chandra Prajapati, Katriina Aalto-Setälä, Akikazu Takada, Shinji Koba, Fumiko Shimizu, Angelos Tsipis



First published in London, United Kingdom, 2020 by IntechOpen
IntechOpen is the global imprint of INTECHOPEN LIMITED, registered in England and Wales, registration number: 11086078, 7th floor, 10 Lower Thames Street, London, EC3R 6AF, United Kingdom
Printed in Croatia

British Library Cataloguing-in-Publication Data
A catalogue record for this book is available from the British Library

Additional hard and PDF copies can be obtained from orders@intechopen.com

Visions of Cardiomyocyte - Fundamental Concepts of Heart Life and Disease
Edited by Angelos Tsipis
p. cm.
Print ISBN 978-1-78985-555-5
Online ISBN 978-1-78985-556-2
eBook (PDF) ISBN 978-1-78985-929-4

For EU product safety concerns:
IN TECH d.o.o., Prolaz Marije Krucifikse Kozulić 3, 51000 Rijeka, Croatia, info@intechopen.com or visit our website at intechopen.com.

# Meet the editor

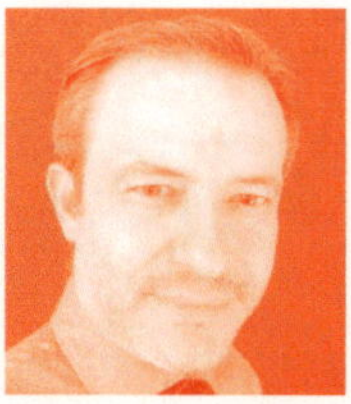

Dr. Angelos Tsipis holds a diploma in medicine (MD) from the Medical School at University "TorVergata," Rome, Italy, and also received a PhD from the National and Kapodistrian University of Athens, Greece. He is a cardiologist at Onassis Cardiac Surgery Center, Athens, Greece, and a research scientist at the First Department of Pathology at the Medical School, University of Athens, Greece. His interests cover cardiomyopathies and specifically cardiovascular pathology and molecular cardiology. He has received six prizes for best research achievement at international and national congresses. Dr. Tsipis has published more than 120 scientific papers in international and national journals and conference proceedings, and edited two monographs and textbooks. He is a member of the editorial board of six scientific journals, a reviewer of 10 journals, and a member of international and national medical societies.

# Contents

**Preface** **XI**

**Section 1**
Myocardial Ischemia **1**

**Chapter 1** **3**
Introductory Chapter: Cardiomyocyte - Fundamental Unit of Heart Life and Disease
*by Angelos Tsipis*

**Chapter 2** **7**
Right Heart Adaptation to Left Ventricular STEMI in Rats
*by Rolf Schreckenberg and Klaus-Dieter Schlüter*

**Chapter 3** **21**
Myocardial Infarction and Circadian Rhythm
*by Ivana Škrlec, Svjetlana Marić and Aleksandar Včev*

**Section 2**
Myocardial Genetics **37**

**Chapter 4** **39**
Current Pathophysiological and Genetic Aspects of Dilated Cardiomyopathy
*by Deborah P. Schild, Sascha I. Ricciardi, Jens G. Hellige, Rolf Vogel and Nisha Arenja*

**Chapter 5** **63**
Modelling of Genetic Cardiac Diseases
*by Chandra Prajapati and Katriina Aalto-Setälä*

**Section 3**
Myocardial Metabolics **85**

**Chapter 6** **87**
Obesity-Related Myocardiopathy
*by Marco Antonio Lopez Hernandez*

**Chapter 7** **99**
Roles of Trans and ω Fatty Acids in Health; Special References to Their Differences between Japanese and American Old Men
*by Akikazu Takada, Fumiko Shimizu and Shinji Koba*

# Preface

The study of the structure and behavior of cardiomyocyte is fundamental to the education of all cardiologists because it is the bridge leading from basic science to clinical cardiology. The marked diversity of cells constituting the tissues and organs of the human body is known. There are more than 200 morphologically distinct adult cell types and this large number reflects the diversity of their function. However, despite this diversity of structure and function, there is a small range of structural subunits and organelles that comprise these cell types. A cell with a particular function will have a predictable constellation of organelles relating to that specialization. So, understanding the structure and function of normal heart cells lays the foundation for developing studies designed to explore the pathogenesis of diseased myocardium. Knowledge of the pathological basis of disease, with particular reference to causation, pathogenesis, and possible natural histories, is essential if the clinical manifestations of disease are to be interpreted and treated in a rational way.

Many pathological states can be represented as expression of disturbances in a normal dynamic equilibrium. Myocardial ischemia may represent a condition if the blood supply to the myocardium does not meet the demand. The energy requirements of heart muscle are high. If this disturbance in the normal equilibrium persists, it triggers a cascade of cellular, inflammatory, and biochemical events, leading to the death of cardiomyocytes. Contraction of cardiomyocytes and the maintenance of their membrane integrity require large amounts of energy. Heart muscle is poorly supplied with endogenous fuel stores, is well vascularized, and is highly aerobic in its metabolism. Interruptions to the blood supply of the myocardium, even for comparatively shorts periods, produce catastrophic results.

Generation, reception, and transduction of signals at an appropriate level are intrinsic to normal cell behavior. Serious functional disturbances may arise when the cells cannot generate or transport an appropriate signal or lack the appropriate receptors to receive an important signal. Intercellular communication is fundamental for normal cardiac function. Synchronization of mechanical and electrical activity is essential to transform the work of individual myocytes into the pumping function of the organ. Desmosome is a specialized adhesive junction that interacts with the cytoskeleton and creates interactions with gap and adherens junctions. Mutations in components of the desmosome lead to a variety of disorders such as arrhythmogenic cardiomyopathy, a disease that bridges the gap between inherited arrhythmia syndromes and heart muscle disorders.

In the introductory chapter, the author discusses the importance of understanding the molecular and cellular basis of cardiovascular disease. Knowledge of the pathological basis of disease with the integration of multilevel biological data and the connection with the clinical practice reveal the potential of personalized medicine, with future implications for prognosis, diagnosis, and management of cardiovascular diseases.

The authors of the second chapter investigate the molecular adaptation of right ventricular (RV) in response to left ventricular (LV) infarction. RV failure is common in patients with acute ST-segment elevated myocardial infarction and animal models of remodeling post-myocardial infarction. However, a systematic analysis of chamber-specific changes in the expression of genes linked to cardiac function, apoptosis, fibrosis, receptor responsiveness, and inflammation is lacking. The underlying reason for biventricular failure due to myocardial infarction and/or transient ischemic events is not clear but may be a consequence of hemodynamic changes during infarction and ischemic events in the RV as well. Nevertheless, RV failure is a severe complication during the subsequent post-infarct period and a limitation to further prognosis.

Human physiological activity and condition during illness are under the control of the circadian rhythm. It is well known that many cardiovascular processes show daily variations depending on the circadian rhythm (blood pressure, heart rate), and the gene expression of the cardiomyocyte circadian clock influences myocardial contractile function, metabolism, and other gene expressions. The authors present a review of the latest knowledge on the impact of circadian rhythm and circadian rhythm genes on myocardial infarction.

The authors of the next chapter discuss the importance of human-induced pluripotent stem cell-derived cardiomyocytes (hiPSC-CMs) to investigate the mutation-specific mechanism. While animal models fail to recapitulate human cardiac disease phenotype properly, hiPSC-CMs have been successful in recapitulating crucial phenotypes of many genetic cardiac diseases in terms of morphology, contractility, $Ca^{2+}$ handling, ion channel biophysics, cell signaling, and metabolism. Most strikingly, hiPSC-CMs provide the patient-specific platform to study the disease mechanism and drug response individually, which the traditional disease modeling technique would never offer. In addition, cardiac subtype-specific arrhythmias and drug screening could be performed with the help of an unlimited supply of hiPSC-CMs, thus chamber-specific treatment modalities could be identified. Certainly, by improving the current weaknesses of hiPSC-CMs, and incorporating with new gene-editing techniques, complex cardiac disease mechanisms could be deciphered and novel effective treatment therapies could be identified to improve the life of cardiac patients.

In the last decades, major advances have been made in the understanding of molecular and genetic issues, as well as in the pathophysiology and clinical assessment of cardiomyopathies. Especially, understanding the genetic basis of dilated cardiomyopathy (DCM) has improved considerably with the availability of genetic analysis. To further improve the prognosis of patients, it is important to regularly gather knowledge about the current state of DCM and adapt the appropriate diagnostic workups. Therefore, this chapter provides the reader with a comprehensive overview of the current state of DCM from definition over etiology, including the genetic aspects to management for cardiovascular specialists.

The following chapter is a review of myocardial changes associated with obesity. It is recognized that obesity contributes to cardiovascular and metabolic disorders through alterations in the levels of adipocyte-derived cytokines called adipokines. The authors conclude that, "our understanding of adipokine biology and obesity-induced adiposopathy increases, and the major challenge will reside in translating this information into new prognostic and therapeutic approaches to limit cardiovascular risk in obese individuals."

Higher intakes of industrially produced trans-fatty acids (IP-TFAs) and of saturated fatty acids are associated with increased risk for congenital heart disease (CHD), and higher intakes of both the ω6 (n-6) polyunsaturated fatty acids (PUFAs) and the omega-3 PUFAs are associated with a lower risk of CHD. Since estimation of dietary intakes of fatty acids (FAs) using questionnaires is challenging (because of out-of-date databases, reliance on memory, poor estimation of portion sizes, etc.), many researchers have begun to measure plasma/blood levels of FAs as more objective biomarkers of exposure. The two general classes of FAs for which biomarkers are most strongly linked with intakes are PUFAs (especially the omega-3 class) and IP-TFAs. Because risk for CHD is much lower in Japan than in the USA, the authors undertook this study to compare the FA profiles in Japanese and American men over the age of 50.

I wish to thank the authors who have contributed so generously to this book. They are all experts in their fields of interest, but have taken time to write on their subjects to make this work as comprehensive as possible.

**Angelos Tsipis, MD, PhD, MSc**
Department of Cardiology,
Onassis Cardiac Surgery Centre,
Athens, Greece

Department of Pathology,
Medical School,
National and Kapodistrian University of Athens,
Athens, Greece

Section 1

# Myocardial Ischemia

Chapter 1

# Introductory Chapter: Cardiomyocyte - Fundamental Unit of Heart Life and Disease

*Angelos Tsipis*

## 1. Introduction

In the field of cardiology, some of the most dramatic advances in recent years have come from understanding the molecular and cellular basis of cardiovascular disease. The knowledge of the pathological basis of disease in some cases allows the development of new strategies for prevention and treatment. This book was planned not only to convey the new facts of cardiovascular diseases but also to boost the excitement and challenges of research in the dynamic area of modern molecular and cellular biology of cardiology.

## 2. Cardiomyocyte: structure and function

Cells are the fundamental unit of life, and the large number of them reflects the diversity of their function. The myocardium is composed principally of specialized muscle cells called cardiomyocytes. The major components of cardiac myocytes, cell membrane (sarcolemma) and T-tubules, necessary in excitation-contraction coupling, thereby facilitate a fast and synchronous contraction across the entire cell volume, sarcoplasmic reticulum, nucleus, and contractile elements. Cardiomyocytes contain many more mitochondria than skeletal muscle cells reflecting the dependence of cardiac muscle cell on aerobic metabolism. The functional intracellular contractile unit of cardiac muscle is the sarcomere that contains the contractile proteins myosin and actin. Sarcomeres also contain the regulatory proteins troponin and tropomyosin. Functional integration of myocytes is mediated by intercalated disks, which join individual cells and within which specialized intercellular junctions permit mechanical and electrical coupling. Intercalated disk contains various junctional complexes including the zonula adherens, desmosomes, and gap junctions. One of the most important types of adhesive interactions required for the formation and maintenance of tissues is that mediated by the cadherin family. The expression and distribution of many of these junctional components are often perturbed in cardiovascular disease [1–4]. One of the components of intercalated disks is gap junctions which facilitate synchronous myocyte contraction by providing electrical coupling. Deregulation of gap junction in cardiovascular disease may contribute to electromechanical dysfunction and arrhythmias. In addition, the cardiac conduction system consists of specialized myocardial fibers that conduct electrical impulses more readily than surrounding myocardial fibers and regulate the rate and the rhythm of the heart.



IntechOpen

## 3. Cardiomyocyte: the basis of life and cardiac disease

The etiology of heart failure involves the interaction of multiple parameters, such as genetic predisposition, environment factors, and chance. Research advances and clinical investigations recognized familial transmission for many cardiomyopathies and confirmed the hypothesis that cardiomyopathies are characterized as *genetic disorders*. Numerous theories regarding the cause of idiopathic dilatative cardiomyopathy have been proposed such as viral myocarditis, autoimmune response against myocardial epitopes, and genetic factors that appear to be more important than previously believed. Nowadays, studies based on a more careful evaluation of disease inheritance and on prospective systematic family screening revealed a high frequency of genetic transmission of the disease in different populations. However, the true frequency is probably still underestimated due to the absence of early markers of the disease and reduced penetrance. Mutations in several known genes including those encoding dystrophin, δ-sarcoglycan, troponin T, β-myosin heavy chain, actin, lamin A/C, and desmin have been identified as a cause of a phenotype [3, 5, 6].

Cells are poised between survival and apoptosis, and their fate rests on a balance of powerful intracellular and extracellular forces, whose signals constantly act upon and counteract each other. In many circumstances, apoptosis is a self-protective programmed mechanism that leads to the suicide of a cell when its survival is deemed detrimental to the organism. In other instances, apoptosis is a pathological process that contributes to many disorders. Although increasing experiment data suggest that necrosis and apoptosis occur in heart failure, the relation between the two conditions and the relevant pathophysiological mechanism are less clear. Significant progress has been made in demonstrating the role of apoptosis in various heart diseases and in elucidating the molecular mechanisms of cardiac apoptosis. The progressive loss of cardiac myocytes is one of the most important pathogenic components of the heart failure. Even though the rate of apoptosis in heart failure is relatively low in absolute numbers, it is significantly higher than that in the normal heart, which has essentially negligible baseline apoptosis. Recently, animal models of heart failure incorporating transgenic technology have confirmed that myocyte apoptosis itself is sufficient to induce heart failure. The elevated presence of p53, Bax, and Bak-positive cells in dilated cardiomyopathy is associated with progressive loss of myocytes in heart failure. On the other hand, increased expression of the antiapoptotic protein bcl-2 in the human myocardium with dilated cardiomyopathy may be a compensation for the loss of myocytes and a possible compensatory antiapoptotic mechanism in the diseased group. Furthermore, the elevated expression of proapoptotic proteins is associated with the progressive loss of myocytes by apoptosis and may play a role in the evolution of the chronic heart failure in patients with old myocardial infarction and chronic ischemic disease. Immunohistochemistry of proapoptotic Bax and antiapoptotic bcl-2 protein demonstrated higher levels of both of these proteins in the diseased group of patients with acute myocardial infarction than normal hearts. A 1.3- and twofold increase in Bax and bcl-2 positive samples was observed in diseased group with acute myocardial infarction compared with the control group. The increased expression of antiapoptotic proteins in acute myocardial infarction represents a possible compensatory mechanism of salvaged myocytes. The prevalence of the apoptotic mechanism or this compensatory antiapoptotic may influence the evolution of heart failure in heart diseases. Thus, the pharmacological manipulation of apoptosis represents an active frontier of drug development [7].

Cell and molecular biology is a rapidly growing field of research and transfers knowledge, from basic cardiology science and preclinical studies, to the clinical cardiology. At the present time, cell priming, bio-nanotechnology, and tissue engineering are coming up as valuable techniques for cell- and tissue-based therapy application in clinical cardiology. The integration of multilevel biological data and the connection with the clinical practice reveal the potential of personalized medicine and future implications for prognosis, diagnosis, and management of cardiovascular diseases.

## Author details

Angelos Tsipis[1,2]

1 Department of Cardiology, Onassis Cardiac Surgery Centre, Athens, Greece

2 Department of Pathology, Medical School, National and Kapodistrian University of Athens, Athens, Greece

*Address all correspondence to: angelostsipis@gmail.com

## References

[1] Cooper GM. The Cell. A Molecular Approach. USA: Sinauer Associates Inc.; 1997. pp. 1-15

[2] Kumar V, Abbas AK, Fausto N. Robbins and Cotran: Pathologic Basis of Disease. 7th ed. Philadelphia: Elsevier Saunders; 2005. pp. 555-557

[3] Tsipis A, Athanassiadou AM, Athanassiadou P, Kavantzas N, Agrogiannis G, Patsouris E. Apoptosis-related factors p53, bcl-2 and the defects of force transmission in dilated cardiomyopathy. Pathology, Research and Practice. 2010;**206**(9):625-630

[4] Kostetskii I, Li J, Xiong Y, Zhou R, Ferrari VA, Patel VV, et al. Induced deletion of the N-cadherin gene in the heart leads to dissolution of the intercalated disc structure. Circulation Research. 2005;**96**(3):346-354

[5] Rubin E, Gorstein F, Rubin R, Schwarting R, Strayer D. Rubin's Pathology: Clinicopathologic Foundations of Medicine. 4th ed. Philadelphia: Lippincott Williams & Wilkins; 2005. pp. 566-570

[6] Mestroni L, Rocco C, Gregori D. Familial dilated cardiomyopathy: Evidence for genetic and phenotypic heterogeneity. Journal of the American College of Cardiology. 1999;**34**(1):181-190

[7] Tsipis A. Heart Muscle and Apoptosis, Cardiomyopathies - From Basic Research to Clinical Management, Josef Veselka. IntechOpen; 2012. pp. 185-198. DOI: 10.5772/29360. Available from: https://www.intechopen.com

Chapter 2

# Right Heart Adaptation to Left Ventricular STEMI in Rats

*Rolf Schreckenberg and Klaus-Dieter Schlüter*

## Abstract

Development of right ventricular (RV) failure in patients after ST-segment elevation myocardial infarction (STEMI) is common. However, a systematic analysis of chamber-specific changes in the expression of genes linked to cardiac function, apoptosis, fibrosis, receptor responsiveness, and inflammation is lacking. Postischemic remodeling was analyzed in rats that received STEMI in the closed chest mode. Rats were sacrificed at day 1, 3, 7, and 120 after surgery. The mRNA expression of genes was quantified by a real-time RT-PCR. Echocardiography was performed after 120 days. Organ weights and systemic blood pressure were determined in addition. Rats developed left and RV dysfunction within 7 days after ischemia/reperfusion and this lasted until the end of the experiments. However, adaptation to ischemia/reperfusion differed significantly between both ventricles. In the LV, a high expression of MMP12, a neutrophile-specific elastase, indicated a significant inflammatory responsiveness that did not occur in RV. A number of differentially regulated genes in the RV exceeded that of the LV at day 3. Postinfarction RV failure is common in rats with ischemia/reperfusion of the left arterial descending aorta. It is associated with severe RV remodeling that occurred delayed to that of the LV. Changes in RV are independent of the initial inflammation.

**Keywords:** myocardial infarction, cardiac remodeling, right heart failure, inflammation, reperfusion injury

## 1. Introduction

Right ventricular (RV) failure is common in patients with acute ST-segment elevated myocardial infarction (STEMI) and animal models of remodeling post-myocardial infarction [1–3]. The underlying reason for biventricular failure due to myocardial infarction and/or transient ischemic events is not clear but may be a consequence of hemodynamic changes during infarction and ischemic events in the RV as well. Nevertheless, RV failure is a severe complication during the subsequent postinfarct period and a limitation of further prognosis [4]. Therefore, it is important to understand the molecular adaptation of the RV in response to LV infarction.

Molecular and cellular mechanisms involved in cardiac remodeling after myocardial infarction are triggered by transcriptional regulation of genes linked to apoptosis, fibrosis, inflammation, calcium handling, and receptor responsiveness. Some of these adaptive mechanisms occur early after reperfusion and activation of the transcription factor AP-1 have been identified as main factors [5]. However, steady-state mRNA levels depend also from RNA degradation leading to a decrease in the expression of some genes. Thus, steady-state mRNA expression of genes involved in cardiac remodeling can be increased or decreased. Real-time RT-PCR allows quantification of such molecular and cellular adaptation in tissues and can be used to characterize such changes in a time- and organ-specific manner. This study was aimed to identify differentially regulated cardiac genes in the LV and RV that are involved in cardiac remodeling during postmyocardial infarction.

The left anterior descending coronary artery was occluded in rats for 45 min and subsequently reopened. Success of occlusion and reperfusion was monitored by ECG recordings. Rats were sacrificed after 1, 3, 7, and 120 days and the left and right ventricles were removed and analyzed thereafter. The hemodynamic consequences were recorded by echocardiography.

## 2. Material and methods

### 2.1 Animal models and animal handling

The investigation conforms to the directive 2010/63/EU of the European Parliament. Use of animals was registered at the Justus-Liebig-University (registration-no.: 417-M). The experimental protocols were approved by the ethics committee for animal experimentation of the local authorities in Giessen, Germany and Szeged, Hungary.

Myocardial infarction and reperfusion was performed in the closed-chest model. To achieve this, rats were anesthetized by inhalation of isoflurane (induction: 5%, maintenance: 2–3%), intubated, and placed on a respirator during surgery to maintain ventilation. Before surgery, 0.03 mg/kg nalbuphine (Nalbuphin Orpha, AOP Orpha Pharmaceuticals, Vienna, Austria) was injected (i.p.). The adequacy of anesthesia was monitored by electrocardiography and pulse rate. A suture was placed around the left anterior descending coronary artery (LAD) and remained subcutaneously [6]. Two hours after the wound closing, 0.03 mg/kg nalbuphine was repeated to alleviate postoperative pain. Seven days later, rats were anesthetized as before and the suture was mobilized and the LAD was occluded for 30 min. The occlusion was monitored by electrocardiography (ST elevation; see **Figure 1**). Thereafter, the occluder was opened again and the suture was cut and the skin was closed in one layer. Sham rats received the same protocol but the occluder was not mobilized after 7 days. Please note that this study is a second end-point analysis of tissue material also used before to characterize the role of arginase in ischemia/reperfusion injury [7].

### 2.2 *Ex vivo* analysis of cardiac function

In order to analyze the cardiac function *ex vivo*, rats were anesthetized again by isoflurane and killed by cervical dislocation. Thereafter, hearts were rapidly excised and the aorta was cannulated for retrograde perfusion with a 16-gauge needle connected to a Langendorff perfusion system. Left ventricular function was determined by insertion of a water-filled balloon into the left ventricle as described before [8]. Hearts were paced during measurements.

### 2.3 In vivo analysis of cardiac function

Transthoracic echocardiography was performed as described previously [9] under isoflurane anesthesia (1.5%) at 120 days after ischemia/reperfusion. Briefly, two-dimensional and M-mode echocardiographic examinations were performed in accordance with the criteria of the American Society of Echocardiography with

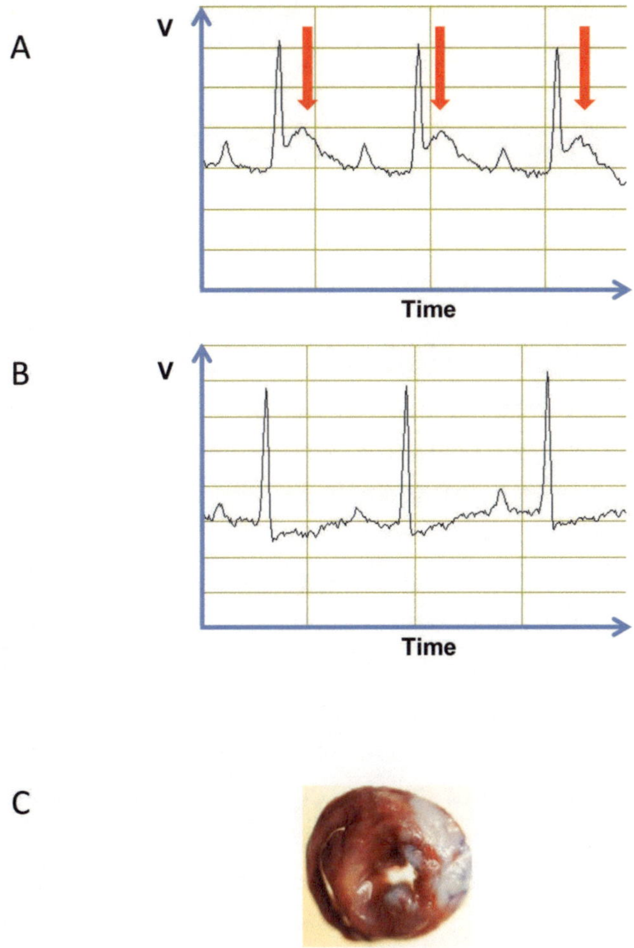


**Figure 1.**
*ECG recording during ischemia (A) and after reperfusion (B) indicating ST elevation in these rats (red arrow). (C) TTC staining visualizing the location of the infarct.*

a Vivid 7 dimension ultrasound system (General Electric Medical Systems) using a phased array 5.5–12 MHz transducer (10S probe). Data of three consecutive heart cycles were analyzed (EchoPac Dimension software; General Electric Medical Systems) by an experienced investigator in a blinded manner. The mean values of three measurements were calculated and used for statistical evaluation. Functional parameters including left ventricular ejection fraction (EF) and fractional shortening (FS) were calculated on four-chamber view images.

## 2.4 qRT-PCR

After removing the hearts from the Langendorff apparatus, the ventricular tissue was carefully isolated and quickly frozen into fluid nitrogen. Tissue samples were prepared to analyze the steady-state mRNA levels of proteins of interest according to the previously described method [8]. Briefly, total RNA was isolated from the ventricles using peqGoldTriFast (peqlab, Biotechnology GmbH, Germany) according to the manufacturer's protocol. To remove genomic DNA contamination, isolated RNA samples were treated with 1 U DNase per mg RNA (Invitrogen, Karlsruhe, Germany) for 15 min at 37°C. One microgram of total RNA was used in 10 μl reaction to synthesize cDNA using superscript RNaseH

| | **Forward** | **Reverse** |
|---|---|---|
| ANP | ATG GGC TCC TTC TCC ATC AC | TCT TCG GTA CCG GAA GCT |
| BNP | ATG ATT CTG CTC CTG CTT TTC | TCT GCA TCG TGG ATT GTT CTG |
| MHC-α | CAC CCT GGA GGA CCA GAT TA | TGG ATC CTG ATG AAC TTC CC |
| TGF-$\beta_1$ | ATT CCT GGC GTT ACC TTG G | CCT GTA TTC CGT CTC CTT GG |
| Biglycan | TGA TTG AGA ATG GGA GCC TGA G | CCT TGG TGA TGT TGT TGG AGT G |
| Decorin | GGC AGT CTG GCT AAT GTT C | CTT CGG AGA TGT TGT TGT TAT G |
| Collagen-1 | GCG AAC AAG GTG ACA GAG | CCA GGA GAA CCA GCA GAG |
| Collagen-3 | TGG AGT CGG AGG AAT G | GCC AGA TGG ACC AAT AG |
| Elastin | TGC TAC TGC TTG GTG GAG AAT G | CGT GGC TGC TGC TGT CTG |
| Fibronectin | TGG AGC AAG AAG GAC AAC | CGG ACA TCT GTG AAG GAG |
| Laminin | CGA GGA TGT CAG CGT TGT | TCA CAG CCG TCT CCA GTC |
| SERCA2a | CGA GTT GAA CCT TCC CAC AA | AGG AGA TGA GGT AGC GGA TGA A |
| Phospholamban | TAT GTC TGC TGC TGA TAT GC | ACT CTT AAA TCG TGA CCC TTC |
| NCX | CGC TAA TCA GCA TTT CAG AG | GCC AGG TTC GTC TTC TTA AT |
| Bax | ACT AAA GTG CCC GAG CTG ATC CAC | TGT CTG CCA TGT GGG G |
| Bcl-2 | ATC TTC TCC TTC CAG CCT GA | TCA GTC ATC CAC AGA GCG AT |
| ODC | GAA GAT GAG TCA AAC GAG CA | AGT AGA TGT TTG GCC TCT GG |
| Arginase-2 | TGA GGA GCA GCG TCT CCC GT | GCT TCT CGG ATG GCG GCT GG |
| eNOS | AGC CCG GGA CTT CAT CAA TCA G | GCC CCA AAC ACC AGC TCA CTC TC |
| Intermedin | TGC CTC AGG GTG GTG GCT CAA CT | GTG GGG GCT GCT GGG AT |
| RAMP-1 | AGC ATC CTC TGC CCT TTC ATT | GAC CAC CAG GGC AGT CAT G |
| RAMP-2 | GCA GCC TAC CTT CTC CGA TCC | TCC TCC ACA CCA CAA GCG TAA C |
| RAMP-3 | CAA CCT GTC GGA GTT CAT CGT | TGT CTC CAT CTC CGT GCA GTT |
| MMP9 | CAA TCC TTG CAA TGT GGA TG | AAA TCT TCT TGG ACT GCG GA |
| MMP12 | TGC AGC TGT CTT TGA TCC AC | GCA TCA ATT TTT GGC CTG AT |
| iNOS | AAG AGA CGC ACA GGC AGA G | CAG CAG GCA CAC GCA ATG |
| Nrf-1 | GGC ATC ACT GGC AGA GGC CG | GCT GCT GCG GTT TCC CCA GA |
| PGC-1α | AGT GCT CAG CCG AGG ACA CGA | TGC CCC TGC CAG TCA CAG GA |
| SDF-1α | CCA AGG TCG TCG CCG TGC TG | GGC TCT GGC GAC ATG GCT CT |
| VEGF | TGC CCC TAA TGC GGT GTG CG | GGC TCA CAG TGA ACG CTC CAG G |
| GATA4 | CTA TGG CCG CCA ACC ACG GG | CGC GGA GTG GGC ACG TAG AC |
| Mef-2c | CAG TTG GGA GAC CGT ACC AC | GTG AGT CCA ATG GGG GAG TG |
| Nkx.2a | CAC ACG CCC TCC TCA GTC AA | GAG TAG CCG TCC GGC TTG AA |
| vWF | AAG ATG GCA AGA GAG TGG GC | CCG TAG GCC TCA CTG GAA AG |
| VE-cadherin | CCA GAA TTT GCC CAG CCC TA | GTC CTC GTT CTT CAG GGC AA |
| B2M | GCC GTC GTG CTT GCC ATT C | CTG AGG TGG GTG GAA CTG AGA C |
| HPRT | CCA GCG TCG TGA TTA GTG AT | CAA GTC TTT CAG TCC TGT CC |

**Table 1.**
*List of primers used in this study.*

reverse transcriptase (200 U/μg; Invitrogen) and oligo dTs (Roche, Mannheim, Germany) as primers. Reverse transcriptase reactions were performed for 60 min at 37°C. Real-time PCR was performed using the Icycler IQ detection system (Bio-Rad, Munich, Germany) in combination with IQ SYBR Green real-time supermix (Bio-Rad). A complete list of all primers used in this study is given in **Table 1**. Data are normalized to hypoxanthine phosphoribosyltransferase (HPRT) expression that was used as a house-keeping gene in this study. Preliminary experiments with β2 microglobulin, which was alternatively considered as house-keeping gene, revealed similar results but higher variability. The relative change in expression was quantified by the ΔΔC method [10].

### 2.5 Statistics

The results are expressed as means ± S.E.M or median with 25 and 75% quartiles as indicated in the legend to the figures. Statistical comparisons were performed by two-side T-Test or Mann-Whitney Test. Levene test was used to check the normal distribution of the samples. A p value of 0.05 was considered as statistical significant.

## 3. Results

### 3.1 Weight of organs, left ventricular pressures, and biventricular functions analysis over time

Body weight, LV weight, RV weight, lung wet weight, and kidney weight increased during the 4-months observation period in sham rats and those undergoing ischemia/reperfusion (**Table 2**). Mean increase in body weight at day 3 after the ischemic event was smaller in the surgery group (+2 g) versus the sham group (+13 g) indicating a small impact of the surgery on general behavior. Differences between both groups in ventricular weight occurred only for the RV at day 1 (**Table 1**). RV weights of rats in the experimental group normalized thereafter. No differences were obtained for lung and kidney weights (**Table 2**). Necrotic tissue was nearly exclusively seen in LV (**Figure 1**).

LV function was determined in vitro. Immediately after ischemia/reperfusion, a significant decline in cardiac function was observed but this was normalized thereafter (**Table 3**). Biventricular function was analyzed after 120 days via echocardiography. RV fractional area change (four-chamber view) and LV ejection fraction (longitudinal four-chamber view) were significantly lower in rats of the experimental group compared to shams (**Table 4**).

### 3.2 Biventricular gene regulation over time

In total, biventricular expression of 36 genes was analyzed by a real-time RT-PCR. These genes cover the following area of interest: cardiac hypertrophy (ANP, BNP, MHC-α), fibrosis (TGF-$\beta_1$, biglycan, decorin, collagen-1, collagen-3, elastin, fibronectin, laminin, MMP9), intracellular calcium handling (SERCA2a, phospholamban, NCX), apoptosis (bax, bcl-2), arginine metabolism (ODC, arginase-2, eNOS), receptor coupling (intermedin, RAMP-1, -2, -3), inflammation (iNOS, MMP12), cardiac metabolism (Nrf-1, PGC-1α), stem cell mobilization (SDF-1α, CXCR4, VEGF), cardiac transcription factors (GATA-4, Mef-2c, Nkx.2a), and endothelial markers (von Willebrand factor (vWF), VE-cadherin). **Figure 2** shows how many of these 36 genes were either

| | BW (g) | LV/BW (mg/g) | RV/BW (mg/g) | Lung/BW (mg/g) | Kidney/BW (mg/g) |
|---|---|---|---|---|---|
| Day 1 | | | | | |
| Sham | 208 ± 28 | 2.76 ± 0.37 | 0.48 ± 0.10 | 8.38 ± 2.06 | 5.87 ± 0.65 |
| I/R | 209 ± 16 | 2.87 ± 0.16 | 0.66 ± 0.07 | 8.90 ± 3.01 | 6.94 ± 2.11 |
| P value | 0.958 | 0.317 | 0.003 | 0.711 | 0.222 |
| Day 3 | | | | | |
| Sham | 222 ± 17 | 2.64 ± 0.11 | 0.57 ± 0.06 | 8.14 ± 2.00 | 6.05 ± 0.39 |
| I/R | 211 ± 21 | 2.69 ± 0.22 | 0.64 ± 0.10 | 7.28 ± 0.77 | 5.77 ± 0.25 |
| P value | 0.292 | 0.550 | 0.135 | 0.674 | 0.133 |
| Day 7 | | | | | |
| Sham | 222 ± 20 | 2.69 ± 0.15 | 0.51 ± 0.08 | 7.47 ± 0.95 | 5.80 ± 0.36 |
| I/R | 225 ± 22 | 2.93 ± 0.25 | 0.51 ± 0.07 | 7.81 ± 1.43 | 6.03 ± 0.61 |
| P value | 0.775 | 0.054 | 1.000 | 0.613 | 0.389 |
| Day 120 | | | | | |
| Sham | 255 ± 16 | 2.69 ± 0.13 | 0.53 ± 0.06 | 8.84 ± 1.81 | 5.85 ± 0.34 |
| I/R | 256 ± 21 | 2.74 ± 0.52 | 0.55 ± 0.12 | 9.89 ± 1.08 | 6.32 ± 0.73 |
| P value | 0.908 | 0.736 | 0.666 | 0.211 | 0.210 |

*Data are means ± S.D. from n = 8–9 rats. Data are given for body weight (BW), left ventricular weight (LV), right ventricular weight (RV), lung weight, and kidney weight. Data for LV, RV, lung, and kidney were normalized to body weight.*

**Table 2.**
*Body weight and organ weight.*

| | Sham | I/R | Δ | P value |
|---|---|---|---|---|
| Day 1 | 157.5 ± 20.9 mmHg | 122.9 ± 21.7 mmHg | Δ = −34.6 mmHg | 0.006 |
| Day 3 | 155.0 ± 23.8 mmHg | 132.0 ± 30.1 mmHg | Δ = −23.0 mmHg | 0.113 |
| Day 7 | 188.2 ± 31.4 mmHg | 162.1 ± 15.4 mmHg | Δ = −26.1 mmHg | 0.054 |
| Day 120 | 144.4 ± 10.4 mmHg | 137.9 ± 22.3 mmHg | Δ = −6.5 mmHg | 0.442 |

*Data are means ± S.D. from n = 8–9 hearts.*

**Table 3.**
*Left ventricular developed pressure (LVDP).*

| | Sham | I/R | Δ | P value |
|---|---|---|---|---|
| LV EF | 65.0 ± 5.8 | 51.3 ± 8.1 | Δ = −13.7% | 0.000 |
| RV FAC | 55.8 ± 7.2 | 45.5 ± 7.2 | Δ = −10.3% | 0.004 |

*Data are means ± S.D. from n = 9–13 rats. LV EF = left ventricular ejection fraction (determined by four-chamber longitudinal view); RV FAC = right ventricular fractional area change (determined by four-chamber view).*

**Table 4.**
*Biventricular function determined by echocardiography.*

upregulated or downregulated in the two ventricles over the time. In general, there was an upregulation of several genes mainly at day 3 postinfarction, whereas a downregulation of genes dominated at days 7 and 120. At the first time point (day 1), there were significant differences in the expression between both ventricles. In the LV, four genes were significantly downregulated: GATA4, VEGF, eNOS, and MHC-α. VEGF, eNOS, and MHC-α genes contain a GATA4 promoter region. As expected, GATA4 expression correlated significantly with that of VEGF, eNOS, and MHC-α (**Figure 3**). Only two genes were upregulated (MMP12, Mef2c) at that time point. As MMP12 is a neutrophil-specific elastase, its strong expression in LV may indicate leukocyte infiltration into the LV during initial tissue repair. In the RV, only one gene was significantly affected by myocardial ischemia/reperfusion at that time (NCX). **Figure 4** shows the relative expression of all genes including those that were either up- or downregulated but without reaching the level of significance. At day 1, there is more variability and, therefore, more transcriptional adaptation in LV compared to RV. In the LV, the strongest downregulation that was not yet significant (>0.05) was found for laminin (again correlated with GATA4; **Figure 3**). The strongest upregulation that was not yet significant was found for MMP9. However, lack of statistical significance for laminin and MMP9 indicates a high interindividual variability. In the RV, ANP and Nkx.2a were strongly upregulated and collagen-3 was strongly downregulated but yet not significant.

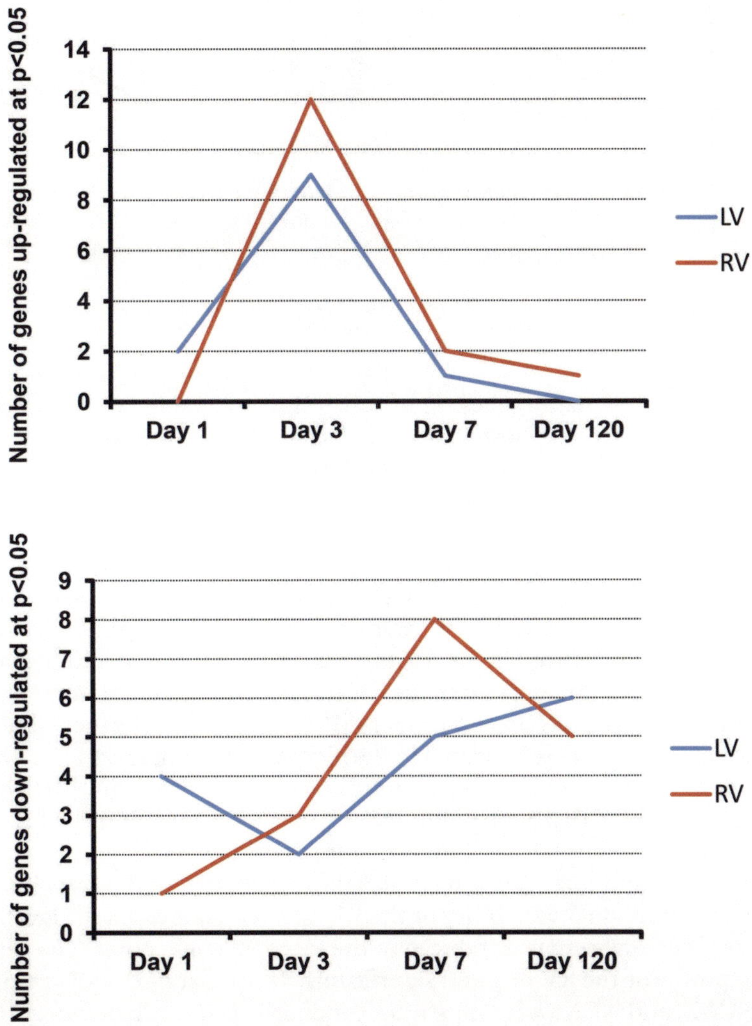


**Figure 2.**
*Time-dependent induction gene regulation in both ventricles. Note that the number of genes differentially regulated (cutoff p < 0.05) is increased in RV after 3 days.*

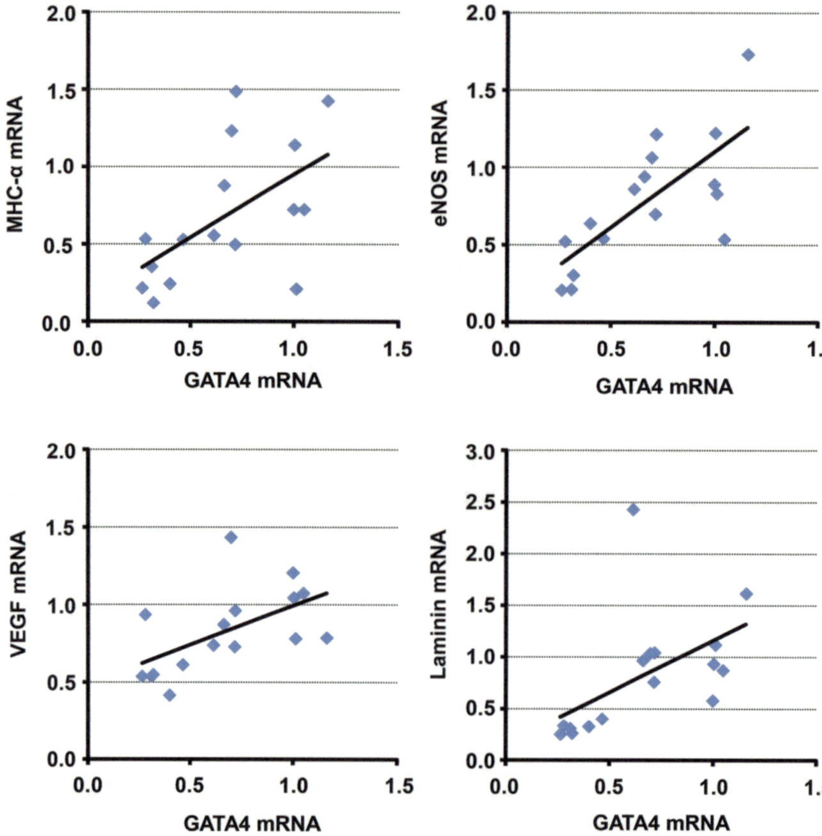


**Figure 3.**
*Correlation between GATA4 expression and that of GATA4-dependent regulated genes.*

At day 3, there were many genes significantly upregulated in both ventricles such as BNP, MHC-α, SERCA2a, phospholamban, NCX, and VEGF. ANP and PGC-1α were also significantly upregulated but in both ventricles. However, the individual variability in RV was strong for these genes so that the level of induction did not reach the level of significance. An exception from the coregulation of genes between both ventricles is the transcription factor Nkx.2a. Nkx2a was upregulated in the LV but beyond the level of detection in the RV. At day 3, only two genes were downregulated in the LV. These are RAMP-2, that was similarly downregulated in the RV and vWF that was slightly reduced in the RV. In addition to the aforementioned genes, six genes were specifically upregulated in the RV that were not induced in the LV. These were decorin, collagen-3, eNOS, RAMP-3, MMP12, and Nrf-1. The increased expression of most of these genes is indicated in the plot shown in **Figure 4.**

At day 7, the expression of most genes induced at early time points was normalized again. However, at that time point, many genes were significantly downregulated. In the LV, this holds for NCX, intermedin, PGC-1α, vWF, and VE-cadherin. Only VE-cadherin and intermedin were also downregulated in the RV; although due to the high individual variability of the RV, this does not reach the level of significance. Only biglycan was induced in the LV at this time point. The gene expression profile of the RV differed significantly from that of the LV at this time point. SERCA2a and NCX were still strongly induced. TGF-β1, bax, bcl-2, RAMP-1, RAMP-2, iNOS, Nrf-1, and CXCR4 were all significantly downregulated. The level of regulation strongly increased the level of regulation of these genes in the left ventricle. **Figure 4** summarizes the expression of all genes at that time point.

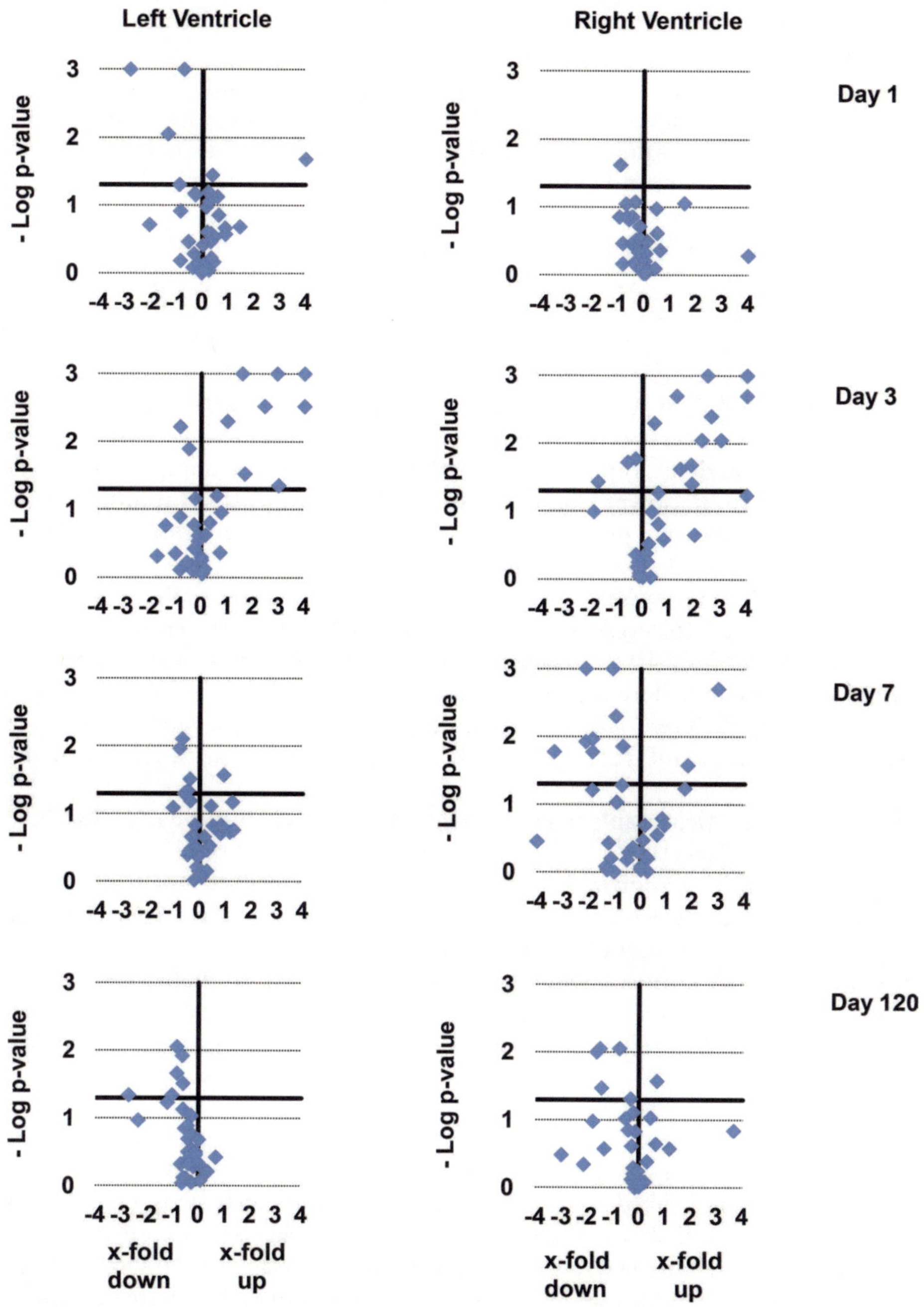


**Figure 4.**
*Profile of gene expression at days 1, 3, 7, and 120 in both ventricles. Upregulated genes are on the right side. Above the horizontal bar differences are below p < 0.05.*

At day 120, 6 out of 36 genes under investigation were downregulated in the LV. These were decorin, RAMP-1, MMP9, MMP12, GATA4, and vWF. Among them, only GATA4 and vWF were not similarly downregulated in the RV. Elastin, fibronectin, bax, and Nkx.2a were specifically downregulated in the RV. Except for Nkx.2a, similar changes (although not significant) were also seen in the LV. The expression of SERCA2a was induced in the RV at that time but not in the LV. Overall, a stronger transcription adaptation is seen in the RV at that time (**Figure 4**).

## 4. Discussion

This study investigated transcriptional adaptation in LV and RV following ischemia/reperfusion in vivo up to 120 days. A higher gene expression level has been attributed to better postinfarct adaptation in female versus male mice [11]. Here, differences were found between both ventricles in the very early phase after ischemia/reperfusion. A significant downregulation of the transcription factor GATA-4 was found specifically in the LV 24 h after reperfusion confirming similar findings after 2 h [11]. According to this observation, the expressions of GATA4-dependent genes (MHC-α, eNOS, and VEGF) were also downregulated. GATA-4 can exert cell survival signaling in cardiac myocytes and delivery of GATA-4 locally to the infarct border zone induces multiple local effects resulting in beneficial remodeling [12, 13]. Regardless of these initial differences, similar changes, mainly induction of gene expression, were found in both ventricles after 3 days. In both ventricles, repression of cardiac gene expression was more prominent rather than induction at later time points, specifically after 4 months. At that time point, the expression profile significantly differed between both ventricles with a more adaptive phenotype in the RV. Again, at this later time point, reduced expression of GATA4 seems to account for some of the differentially downregulated genes in the LV. In summary, this study highlights the differential expression of GATA4 in LV and RV after successful reperfusion and correlates the expression of GATA4 with main differences in molecular adaptation between both ventricles. Regardless of the different molecular adaptation, LV and RV developed a drop of function although the infarct area and inflammation was specifically located at the left ventricle.

The cardiac ventricle is able to respond to ischemic stress with changes in steady-state mRNA levels within 24 h. In principle, steady-state levels of mRNA are the sum of mRNA formation and degradation and the quantification of steady-state levels does not necessarily identify mechanisms that cause these changes. However, in the current study, the main changes in ventricular expression that occurred within 24 h in the LV corresponded to genes that are known to obtain a GATA-4 promoter responsive element. Please note that only the LV is exposed to ischemia/reperfusion. Moreover, GATA-4 itself was also downregulated. It should be noted that within the first few hours after the ischemic event, transcriptional changes were mainly present in the LV.

The response of the heart to LV ischemia and reperfusion significantly differed at day 3. At that time, strong molecular adaptations were obtained in both ventricles. In most cases, these were linked to an upregulation of genes indicating an active adaptation to the postischemic stress. Interestingly, most genes that were upregulated in the LV were also regulated in the RV. An exception to this rule was Nkx.2a. This cardiac-specific transcription factor was below the level of detection in the RV but induced in the LV, probably indicating an active regenerative process. This may indicate cardiac differentiation of cells infiltrated into the infarct-affected ventricle (possibly circulating stem cells), or a cardiac differentiation of cells that were located in the LV and that still have a potential to differentiate (cardiac progenitor cells). Alternatively, it may indicate an active repair process of terminally differentiated cardiomyocytes (hypertrophy). However, the more important finding was the observation that a couple of genes were specifically upregulated in the RV that are not induced in the LV. As such decorin, an endogen inhibitor of the profibrotic cytokine TGF-β1, eNOS, increasing the bioavailability of nitric oxide, and Nrf-1, improving mitochondrial biogenesis, were identified. Each of these factors is a marker of compensatory hypertrophy.

One week after the ischemic event, the initial activation of gene transcription is normalized and replaced by downregulation of many genes in LV and

RV. Interestingly among them are endothelial cell markers and genes linked to cardiac metabolism. Thus, the molecular adaptation switches into a profile of maladaptation. In concert with this view, biglycan, a factor that favors fibrosis, was induced in the LV. In the RV, the expression of profibrotic genes was downregulated as well as the expression of inflammatory markers. Again, the molecular adaptation of the RV seems to be more favorable than that of the LV.

Four months after the ischemic event, the cardiac function was reduced in both ventricles. At that time, decorin was downregulated in both ventricles. Moreover, the RV was characterized by downregulation of elastin and fibronectin. Both molecules are required for a proper cardiac function. In summary, although the molecular adaptation of the RV to LV myocardial infarction differs from that of the LV, the corresponding molecular adaptation of the RV leads to dysfunction of the RV as well.

In this study, we analyzed also the expression of intermedin and the receptor activation modifier proteins (RAMP). They have been analyzed with respect to cardiac regulation in the context of pressure-induced hypertrophy but data on the expression in ischemia and reperfusion are lacking. Intermedin (=adrenomedullin-2) potentially stabilized cardiac function by binding to CGRP receptors that are linked to RAMP-1, -2, or -3. This study shows a downregulation of intermedin in the RV at day 3 and in the LV at day 7. Thus, it is differentially regulated during the subsequent molecular adaptation after ischemia/reperfusion but not as a direct response to the ischemic event itself. Significant downregulation of RAMP-2 and RAMP-1 days after myocardial infarction in both ventricles (RAMP-2) and specifically in the RV (RAMP-1) suggests an impairment of receptor signaling during CGRP-receptors during the subsequent remodeling process. As the development of cardiac dysfunction occurred in both ventricles within 4 months, this observation requires future work because this may be a likely candidate for the subsequent development of heart failure.

Finally, it should be mentioned that this study has of course some limitations. Firstly, data are restricted to genes which mRNA steady-state levels are different between sham and ischemia/reperfusion at a p value of 0.05. This does not exclude the possibility that genes that are strongly regulated but below a p value of 0.05 due to a higher individual variation are not relevant for the molecular adaptation. Secondly, the level of significance is a variable of the n number of animals that are investigated. Here, we used eight rats per group. A lower n reduces the number of genes identified as significantly regulated. However, these limitations are counterbalanced by the quantitative real-time RT-PCR protocol and even more important by the high number of genes under investigation and the analysis of groups of genes linked to specific adaptations (i.e., linked to fibrosis, apoptosis, etc.). This allows a more general view on the adaptation process.

In conclusion, the study identifies a time-dependent difference in the response of LV and RV to STEMI. In the early phase of LV remodeling, GATA-4-dependent downregulation was dominant. The novel and important finding from this study is, however, that a delayed but significant molecular adaptation of the RV. This RV adaptation in the absence of necrosis seems to be more adaptive but still not sufficient to preserve the function. The regulation of RAMP-2 in both ventricles may be one candidate for future research.

## Acknowledgements

We thank Nadine Woitasky and Peter Volk for excellent technical support. The data of this study are in part results of the thesis of Pia Weber.

## Funding

This study was supported by the Deutsche Forschungsgemeinschaft (grants to R. Schulz and K.-D. Schlüter within the graduate school "PROMISE"/IRTG1566, a grant to K.-D. Schlüter (SCHL 324/7-1), a grant to T. Schreckenberg (Deutsche Herzstiftung)). K.-D Schlüter is principal investigator in the CRC 1213 "Pulmonary Hypertension and Cor pulmonale", project B05.

## Author details

Rolf Schreckenberg and Klaus-Dieter Schlüter*
Physiologisches Institut, Justus-Liebig University Giessen, Germany

*Address all correspondence to:
klaus-dieter.schlueter@physiologie.med.uni-giessen.de

## References

[1] Masci PG, Francone M, Desmet W, Ganame J, Todiere G, Donato R, et al. Right ventricular ischmemic injury in patients with acute ST-segment elevation myocardial infarction. Circulation. 2010;**122**:1405-1412

[2] Wei S, Chow LTC, Shum IOL, Qin L, Sanderson JE. Left and right ventricular collagen type I/III ratios and remodeling post-myocardial infarction. Journal of Cardiac Failure. 1999;**5**:117-126

[3] Nahrendorf M, Hu K, Fraccarollo D, Hiller K-H, Haase A, Bauer WR, et al. Time course of right ventricular remodeling in rats with experimental myocardial infarction. American Journal of Physiology. Heart and Circulatory Physiology. 2003;**284**:H241-H248

[4] Mehta SR, Eikelboorn JW, Natarajan MK, Diaz R, Yi C, Gibbons RJ, et al. Impact of right ventricular involvement on mortality and morbidity in patients with inferior myocardial infarction. Journal of the American College of Cardiology. 2001;**37**:37-43

[5] Harpster MH, Bandyopadhyay S, Thomas DP, Ivanov PS, Keele JA, Pineguina N, et al. Earliest changes in left ventricular transcriptome postmyocardial infarction. Mammalian Genome. 2006;**17**:701-715

[6] Bencsik P, Kupai K, Giricz Z, Görbe A, Pipis J, Murlasits Z, et al. Role of iNOS and peroxynitrite-matrix metalloproteinase-2 signaling in myocardial late preconditioning in rats. American Journal of Physiology-Heart and Circulatory Physiology. 2010;**299**:H512-H518

[7] Schreckenberg R, Weber P, Cabrera-Fuentes HA, Steinert I, Preissner KT, Bencsik P, et al. Mechanism and consequences of the shift in cardiac arginine metabolism following ischmaemia and reperfusion in rats. Thrombosis and Haemostasis. 2015;**113**:482-493

[8] da Costa Rebelo RM, Schreckenberg R, Schlüter K-D. Adverse cardiac remodeling in spontaneously hypertensive rats: Acceleration by high aerobic exercise intensity. The Journal of Physiology. 2012;**590**:5389-5400

[9] Kocsis GF, Sárközy M, Bencsik P, Pipicz M, Varga ZV, Pálóczi J, et al. Preconditioning protects the heart in a prolonged uremic condition. American Journal of Physiology-Heart and Circulatory Physiology. 2012;**303**:H1229-H1236

[10] Livak KJ, Schmittgen TD. Analysis of relative gene expression data using real-time quantitative PCR in the 2(-ΔΔCT). Methods. 2001;**25**:402-408

[11] Chen Q, Williams R, Healy CL, Wright CD, Wu SC, O'Connell TD. An association between gene expression and better survival in female mice following myocardial infarction. Journal of Molecular and Cellular Cardiology. 2010;**49**:801-811

[12] Suzuki YJ, Nagase H, Day RM, Das DK. GATA-4 regulation of myocardial survival in the preconditioned heart. Journal of Molecular and Cellular Cardiology. 2004;**37**:1195-1203

[13] Bian J, Popovic ZB, Benejam C, Kiedrowski M, Rodriguez LL, Penn MS. Effect of cell-based intercellular delivery of transcription factor GATA4 on ischemic cardiomyopathy. Circulation Research. 2007;**100**:1626-1633

Chapter 3

# Myocardial Infarction and Circadian Rhythm

*Ivana Škrlec, Svjetlana Marić and Aleksandar Včev*


## Abstract

Human physiological activity and condition during illness are under the control of the circadian rhythm. Circadian rhythms handle a wide diversity of physiological and metabolic functions, and the interruption of these rhythms has been linked to obesity, sleep disorders, metabolic and psychological disorders, and cardiovascular events such as myocardial infarction (MI), stroke, and vascular death. Disruption of circadian rhythms increases the risk of developing myocardial infarction, indicating that circadian genes might play an essential role in determining disease susceptibility. It is well known that many cardiovascular processes show daily variations depending on the circadian rhythm (blood pressure, heart rate), and the gene expression of the cardiomyocyte circadian clock influences myocardial contractile function, metabolism, and other gene expressions. We present a review of the latest knowledge on the impact of circadian rhythm and circadian rhythm genes on myocardial infarction. Today, in a time of personalized medicine, it is essential to know each person's circadian rhythm for its treatment and possible inclusion in the diagnostic procedures.


**Keywords:** cardiomyocytes, circadian rhythm, myocardial infarction

## 1. Introduction

Everyday life is organized according to three different clocks: the solar clock which gives us light and temperature during the day, the social clock which determines the working day, and the biological clock which we notice during shift work or when we adjust to a reduced amount of daylight. In real life, the circadian clock is synchronized within 24 hours of the solar clock [1, 2].

It is known that almost all cardiovascular events occur in a circadian manner with a higher frequency in the morning after waking [3]. In the peripheral clocks of the cardiovascular tissues or cells, there is daily expression of the clock-controlled genes (CCG) synchronized and regulated by central clock [4, 5]. Disturbances of circadian rhythm can lead to cardiovascular disease.

Today we are facing a global epidemic of cardiovascular disease. In 2015 cardiovascular disease was the cause of 17.7 million deaths worldwide or 31% of total mortality. Of these 7.4 million deaths were caused by ischemic heart disease and 6.7 million by cerebrovascular diseases, according to World Health Organization (WHO) [6].

## 2. Circadian rhythm

Circadian rhythm is controlled by a molecular clock located in almost every cell. A hierarchical system organizes molecular clocks—the master clock is located in the suprachiasmatic nucleus (SCN) in the hypothalamus [2, 7], while the peripheral clocks are located in each organ or cell. The central clock regulates physiological functions via the autonomic nervous system, humoral mediators, and other still unknown factors [7, 8]. In the maintenance and generation of circadian or biological rhythm in humans, a whole series of anatomical (suprachiasmatic nucleus), neurological (retinohypothalamic paths) and neuroendocrine (melatonin) systems are involved, indicating that the biology of the circadian rhythm of humans is similar to that of animals [9].

The master clock in the SCN consists of about 100,000 neurons in humans. It is the only molecular clock that receives light as an input signal from the retina. Internal clocks are synchronized with light depending on the time of day. SCN receives a direct light signal from the retina via the optic nerve from the photoreceptor called the intrinsically photoreceptive retinal ganglion cell (ipRGC), which expresses the circadian photopigment, melanopsin [10]. The signal is further transmitted to peripheral clocks via the endocrine system [11, 12]. The central clock synchronizes each of the peripheral clocks in the body, and the primary circadian hormone is melatonin [13]. The pineal gland secretes melatonin during the night. Melatonin plays an essential role in maintaining the circadian rhythm depending on the period of light or darkness. The main difference between the master and peripheral clocks is in their degree of intercellular interaction. Peripheral clocks are under the influence of the master clock from the SCN via hormones, chemical signals and other metabolites (such as food), as well as by changes in the body, such as body temperature [11, 12].

On the other hand, due to the high degree of neuron connection the master clock in the SCN is not under the influence of internal signals but only under the influence of light [14]. Peripheral tissues integrate central clock signals with environmental factors (including sleepiness, physical activity, and feeding) and their autonomic rhythms which regulate the metabolism in a circadian manner [10]. The rhythm of the peripheral clocks in humans is measured by direct measurement of physiological changes, or by determining the expression of the clock genes. Central and peripheral clocks together control the daily circadian rhythm of the metabolism [15].

Feeding time is one of the key triggers or external factors that sets the phases of the peripheral clocks [15]. Complex feedback loops connect the circadian clock with metabolic pathways and integrate these systems independently of light [10]. It is believed that the central clock regulates the metabolism by hormones (primarily cortisol and melatonin) and synaptic signaling (via the autonomic nervous system) [10]. Feeding is a circadian event that serves not only as the output of the central clock, but also as an input signal for peripheral clocks because peripheral tissues communicate with the brain through ghrelin, leptin, glucose, and insulin. Circadian feeding contributes to the interworking of the clock and metabolism, which is crucial for metabolic homeostasis [16]. The central clock rhythm is primarily related to light, whereas peripheral tissue rhythms derive from the input of signals from the central clock, external factors (light, physical activity, feeding, and sleepiness) and the availability of numerous metabolites [15]. All these signals affect the molecular clock, creating a complex correlation between the circadian clock and physiological processes [10]. SCN coordinates all cellular circadian clocks in the organs and tissues through its rhythmic outcomes, to adapt physiology to Earth's rotation [17].

The two clock systems become desynchronized when their drivers or stimuli do not coincide because different stimuli affect the phases of the central and peripheral clocks. This mismatch disrupts the metabolism because the two clock systems coordinate interlinked metabolic pathways. Circadian rhythm mismatch increases the risk of developing metabolic diseases [15].

The central clock is primarily triggered by light, and its rhythm is often measured by determining the concentrations of melatonin, cortisol or body temperature [15]. The expression of the clock genes is disrupted in pathological conditions. Such a change may result in different tissue response to external signals and accelerate tissue damage. The loss of synchronization can lead to various diseases, including an increased incidence of cardiovascular disease [18].

## 3. Molecular basis of circadian rhythm

The central clock genes are expressed in a circadian manner in the SCN, and light is one of the main initiators (so-called *zeitgeber*) and can reset the phase of the rhythm. The first circadian rhythm gene discovered was the *Per* gene in the fruit fly in 1971 [19, 20], while the first circadian rhythm gene discovered in the vertebrae was the *CLOCK* gene [21]. There are about 10 circadian rhythm genes known to regulate cyclic expression of mRNA and protein, via transcription and translation feedback loops [22]. In the SCN there are four essential proteins: ARNTL (Aryl Hydrocarbon Receptor Nuclear Translocator-Like) and CLOCK (Circadian Locomotor Output Cycles Caps) are activators, while PER (Period) and CRY (Cryptochrome) are transcription inhibitors. The feedback of the circadian rhythm gene maintains circadian oscillations in one cell at the transcriptional and posttranscriptional levels, and the transition from light to dark triggers these oscillations. The whole process of activation and repression of gene expression within the loop lasts for about 24 hours. These transcriptional factors trigger numerous physiological changes by acting on the expression of the same genes, and other clock-controlled genes [23, 24].

ARNTL and CLOCK heterodimers bind to regulatory elements of the promoters and enhancers (E-box) of the *PER* and *CRY* genes and stimulate their expression and the expression of other clock-controlled genes. Overnight the amount of PER and CRY proteins gradually increases, and heterodimers are created in the cytoplasm. The phosphorylated PER-CRY heterodimers are translocated into the nucleus where they inhibit the ARNTL-CLOCK protein complex. Therefore, during the day, transcription of *PER* and *CRY* genes is reduced, while the levels of PER and CRY protein decrease due to their degradation by ubiquitin. The PER-CRY heterodimers directly bind to the ARNTL-CLOCK complex, and as PER2 contains histone deacetylase, the chromatin structure changes, resulting in transcription termination. Also, the PER-CRY heterodimer is in interaction with RNA-binding proteins and helicase that are important in stopping transcription independently of the interaction with the ARNTL-CLOCK complex. Additionally, PER-CRY heterodimers regulate the transcription of various nucleic hormone receptors [25–28].

During the day a new cycle begins by the termination of the ARNTL-CLOCK heterodimer inhibition. Casein kinase 1 (CK1) controls the amount of phosphorylation or degradation of PER-CRY heterodimers and thereby determines the amount of PER-CRY heterodimer entering the nucleus and inhibiting the ARNTL-CLOCK complex. CK1 phosphorylates the proteins and thus regulates their activity [29].

The additional negative loop is REV-ERBα that binds to the REV-ERB/ROR response element (RRE) of the *ARNTL* and *CLOCK* genes, and prevents their transcription. Also, RORα (Retinoic Acid Receptor-related Orphan Receptor) binds to the same regulatory elements of the *ARNTL* gene as well as REV-ERBα. With REV-ERBα degradation overnight, RORα promotes transcription of the *ARNTL* gene [30]. The second regulatory loop consists of ARNTL-CLOCK heterodimers which promote the transcription of the nucleic receptors REV-ERBα and RORα [31] (**Figure 1**).

Circadian clock genes have an essential role in many physiological processes. Thus, animal models demonstrate that the *ARNTL* gene plays an essential role in lipid metabolism because it induces the expression of genes involved in lipogenesis in adipose tissue in a circadian manner [32]. Pancreatic beta cells have a circadian clock dependent on ARNTL and CLOCK protein oscillations, which regulate insulin secretion depending on the stage of alertness. Abnormalities of the pancreas clock may trigger the onset of diabetes [33]. It was found that *CLOCK* polymorphisms are associated with body weight, the risk for metabolic syndrome and insomnia in humans [9, 32], and polymorphisms of the *PER2* and *PER3* genes are associated with sleep disorders [34, 35]. Some variants of *CRY1* and *CRY2* genes are associated with metabolic syndrome, particularly hypertension and increased triglyceride levels in the blood [36]. Many variants of the circadian rhythm genes are associated with the risk factors for the development of cardiovascular diseases such as blood pressure, glucose concentration [23, 37]. An overview of the essential circadian rhythm genes with their roles is shown in **Table 1** [38, 39].

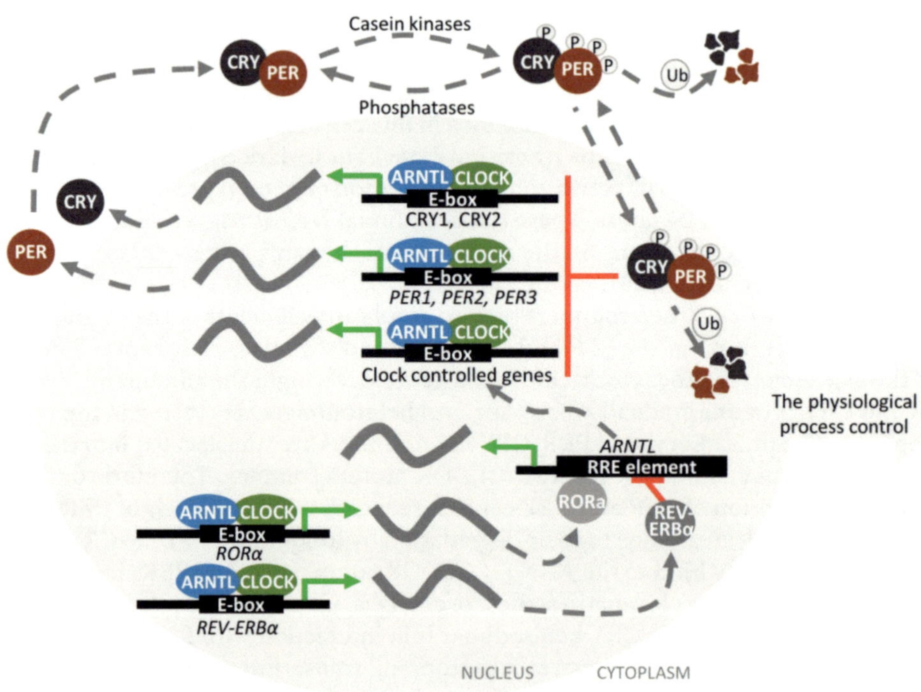


**Figure 1.**
*The molecular mechanism of circadian rhythm in humans. ARNTL and CLOCK activate transcription of CRY and PER, nuclear receptors (REV-ERBα and RORα) and other clock-controlled genes. CRY and PER heterodimerize and phosphorylate by casein kinases and translate into the nucleus where they prevent binding of the ARNTL-CLOCK to the regulatory regions of target genes. In the second feedback loop, REV-ERBα prevents the transcription of ARNTL because it binds to the RRE element, while overnight the same regulatory elements bind RORα and activate transcription of ARNTL. Also, ARNT-CLOCK heterodimers activate transcription of the REV-ERBα and RORα proteins. ARNTL—aryl hydrocarbon receptor nuclear translocator-like, CLOCK—circadian locomotor output cycles kaput, CRY—cryptochrome, PER—period, P—phosphate, RORα—retinoic-related orphan receptor alpha, RRE element—REV-ERB/ROR response element, Ub—ubiquitin.*

| Gene | Function |
|---|---|
| ***ARNTL*** (*Aryl hydrocarbon Receptor Nuclear Translocator-Like*) | Rhythmically expressed. Physically associates with CLOCK. Promotes transcription of *PER* and *CRY*. It is involved in the risk for hypertension, adipogenesis, and glucose metabolism. |
| ***CK1ε*** (*Casein kinase 1 ε*) | Physically associates with and phosphorylates PER. Affects PER stability and nuclear localization. |
| ***CLOCK*** (*Circadian Locomotor Output Cycles Kaput*) | Constitutively expressed. Physically associates with *ARNTL*. Promotes transcription of *PER* and *CRY*. It is involved in the platelet rhythmic activity, response of cardiomyocytes to fatty acids, lipid, and glucose metabolism. |
| ***CRY1*** (*Cryptochrome 1*)<br>***CRY2*** (*Cryptochrome 2*) | Physically associates with and stabilizes PER. Negative regulator of Per and Cry transcription. |
| ***PER1*** (*Period 1*)<br>***PER2*** (*Period 2*)<br>***PER3*** (*Period 3*) | Physically associates with CRY. Positive regulator of *ARNTL*. They are involved in the aortic endothelial function. |
| ***REV-ERBα*** (*nuclear receptor subfamily 1 group D member 1*) | Associates with regulatory elements and negative regulator of the *ARNTL* and *CLOCK* transcription. It is involved in triglyceride and lipid metabolism, and circadian activity of PAI-1. |
| ***RORα*** (*Retinoic-related orphan receptor alpha*) | Associates with regulatory elements and positive regulator of the *ARNTL*. It is involved in lipid metabolism. |
| ***TIM*** (*Timeless*) | Circadian function not known. Physically associates with CRY. Negative regulator of *PER* and *CRY* transcription *in vitro*. |

**Table 1.**
*The essential circadian rhythm genes in mammals.*

Numerous studies on animal models, as well as human populations, have confirmed the association of the circadian clock gene with metabolic syndrome and cardiovascular diseases [15, 40, 41].

## 4. Cardiovascular diseases

The WHO data for 2017 show that cardiovascular diseases were the cause of 19.9 million deaths worldwide, and about 80% of deaths from cardiovascular diseases were due to myocardial infarction and stroke [42]. It is estimated that by 2030, 23.6 million people will die annually due to cardiovascular diseases [43].

Cardiovascular diseases are the primary cause of death in developed countries of the world, and in less developed parts of the world, this mortality is rising and overtaking mortality rates for infectious diseases [44].

There are variable and constant risk factors for cardiovascular disease. The variable risk factors are those that can be affected by therapy and lifestyle change, such as smoking, hyperlipoproteinemia, hypertension, and to some extent diabetes and homocysteinemia. The constant risk factors cannot be affected, namely age, genetic predisposition, gender, and menopause. The general risk factors which can be altered most are smoking, hypertension and hyperlipidemia, and obesity and diabetes whose prevalence has risen in the last few decades. However, some recent risk factors (fibrinogen, lipoprotein (a), homocysteine) should not be ignored. All of these contribute to total cardiovascular risk [45].

Cardiometabolic risk factors are determined by a cluster of metabolic and cardiovascular changes. Diabetes and obesity are also associated with reduced quality of life and increased economic burden on the person and society [46, 47]. Cardiovascular diseases and type 2 diabetes share common pathophysiological mechanisms of insulin resistance and risk factors for cardiovascular diseases, such as metabolic syndrome. Excessive weight plays a significant role because fatty tissue becomes an active endocrine organ that secretes low-level inflammation mediators, and these stimulate the development of metabolic syndrome and vascular diseases [32, 48, 49].

## 5. Myocardial infarction

Myocardial infarction is the leading cause of mortality in developed countries and developing countries. It can be caused and triggered by different pathophysiological processes. Myocardial infarction is an inflammatory disease due to the death of myocardial cells because of complete coronary circulation interruption, which is in most cases a consequence of thrombotic occlusion of the coronary artery at the site of the activated atherosclerotic plaque. An electrocardiogram (ECG) of the ST elevation is only an indirect indicator of the fact that ischemia affects all three layers of cardiac muscle (endocardium, myocardium, and epicardium) [50].

ST-elevation myocardial infarction (STEMI) is the most severe form of acute coronary syndrome. Myocardial infarction is accompanied by increased cellular oxidative stress in the pericardial cavity [51]. The primary cause of infarction is platelet aggregation in the coronary artery. The platelet activity is the highest in the morning. Also, in the morning hours, mental and physical activity increase due to cortisol and catecholamine elevation, which increases cardiac output [45]. The biochemical markers of myocardial damage are cardiac troponin T or troponin I in serum. These biochemical markers are more reliable than those previously used, such as measurement of creatine kinase (CK). The initial increase in troponin in peripheral blood in patients with infarction occurs over 3–4 hours with a permanent increase for up to 2 weeks after infarction. In order to confirm or exclude myocardial damage, troponin T serum levels are repeated in the first 6–12 hours after severe chest pain [52].

The classification of myocardial infarction in five types was introduced in 2007 and established the clinical criteria for its exact differentiation [50]. Type 1 is related to a coronary plaque rupture, fissuring, or dissection with resulting intraluminal thrombosis. Type 2 myocardial infarction is secondary to myocardial ischemia resulting from increased oxygen demand or decreased supply. Type 3 myocardial infarction is linked to unexpected cardiac death when cardiac biomarkers are unavailable. Types 4 and 5 myocardial infarction are procedure related [53].

In the study of Saaby et al., [54] it was shown that the most significant number of patients with myocardial infarction come under Type 1 (72%). In patients with Type 1 myocardial infarction, changes in the ECG are seen either as the elevation or depression of the ST segment; the troponin T level also increases in the blood and serves as a diagnostic marker. The troponin T level in the blood is higher in patients with Type 1 myocardial infarction than Type 2 [55].

For manifestation of infarction, apart from lifestyle, a genetic background of myocardial infarction is also essential. A positive family history of myocardial infarction is a major cardiovascular risk factor [56]. Coronary artery disease and myocardial infarction have a genetic background in 50–60% of cases. Many genes are found in the genetic background of myocardial infarction. Whole genome association studies have revealed many variants of genes associated with increased risk for myocardial infarction [56]. So far the most frequently explored genes with increased risk for myocardial infarction are involved in the metabolic pathways of lipid metabolism and development of type 2 diabetes. The relationship between the circadian rhythm genes and the onset of myocardial infarction will be discussed below.

## 6. Myocardial infarction and circadian rhythm

Many cardiovascular events and diseases have a circadian pattern of appearance. The normal circadian blood pressure shows the two highest values during the day, around 9 am and 7 pm, while there is a slight decrease around 3 pm. It is considered that circadian variations in the tone of coronary vessels and endothelial function play an essential role in the onset of myocardial infarction. As myocardial infarction is significant medical stress, it causes increased cortisol levels in plasma [3]. In the acute phase of myocardial infarction, the phase of the circadian clock in the ischemic part of the heart differs from the non-ischemic part of the heart. The arrhythmia may occur because of the difference in the phase of the rhythm, or different expressions of the circadian clock genes. The loss of synchronization of the circadian rhythm between organs or tissues occurs more often than we would expect [4]. Circadian regulation of physiological processes is regulated locally. Peripheral tissue clocks control tissue-specific expression [27].

Homeostatic changes, gene expression changes, and external triggers can cause a stressful environment and cause damage to the atherosclerotic plaque in the coronary arteries in the morning, when prothrombin is increased [57]. Many intrinsic vasoactive and cardioactive substances, such as angiotensin II, melatonin, plasminogen activator inhibitor 1 (PAI-1), glucocorticoids, epinephrine, norepinephrine, and nitrogen oxide, show a specific circadian pattern. The fibrinolytic system, which regulates PAI-1, shows a circadian pattern of occurrence in both healthy patients and those with ischemic heart disease. The concentration and activity of PAI-1 depend on the circadian rhythm and are the highest in the morning [28]. CLIF (Cycle-Like Factor) expression in endothelial cells creates heterodimers with CLOCK protein, and binds to the E-box of the *PAI-1* gene promoter and promotes its expression, while PER2 and CRY1 inhibit expression of *PAI-1* by blocking heterodimer CLOCK-CLIF. CLIF controls the circadian rhythm of PAI-1 in endothelial cells, which might explain the higher incidence of myocardial infarction in the morning [26, 58]. As a result of this, the fibrinolytic system in patients with MI might be a potential goal for chronotherapy, to treat acute cardiovascular events. The circadian clock regulates the endothelial response to vascular injury. The main factor that can be affected by potential chronotherapy is PAI-1 because it is a crucial fibrinolysis inhibitor [59]. Chronotherapy includes the accurate timing of drug taking and can improve the therapeutic efficacy of the drug, while limiting its toxicity [41]. That is why many studies support chronotherapy for cardiovascular disease by limiting pathogenesis and improving treatment after the occurrence of acute cardiovascular events [59].

It is known that melatonin levels decrease during the night in coronary heart disease and infarction. Melatonin is an antioxidant that can inhibit the action of reactive oxygen radicals during heart ischemia. It also plays a vital role in regulating blood pressure, depending on the circadian rhythm. Animal studies have shown that animals with the pineal gland removed develop hypertension. Clinical examinations have shown that in patients with hypertension melatonin drugs taken daily before bedtime reduced blood pressure [3].

The appearance of myocardial infarction has two peaks during the day. The highest incidence of myocardial infarction is during the morning, and the second peak occurs late at night [60]. The beta blockers prevent increased sympathetic activity, catecholamine concentration, heart rate, blood pressure and lack of oxygen in the heart, and these are the physiological reasons for the existence of two peaks of myocardial infarction [57, 61].

Ischemia occurs in the morning due to increased oxygen demand, whereas in the evening it is due to decreased coronary blood flow. The appearance of myocardial infarction depends on ethnic origin, and the British differ from Asians in the frequency of the infarction [3]. In the Mediterranean, the highest incidence of myocardial infarction is between midday and midnight, while in the UK the highest incidence is between midnight and midday [62]. Numerous factors might affect the later occurrence of infarction in the Mediterranean, such as the number of sunlight hours, inequality in the prevalence of risk factors for cardiovascular disease, and the habit of afternoon rest or 'siesta' [63]. It has also been noted that the incidence of myocardial infarction is higher in the winter [3]. The specific circadian pattern of infarction symptoms has been observed, and the correlation of the circadian rhythm gene with the infarction investigated. The role of the molecular circadian clock in myocardial activity was initially investigated on animal models. It has been observed that the clock gene mutations of the circadian rhythm affect the heart rate, myocardial contractility, energy metabolism, which altogether leads to ischemia [64, 65]. In contrast, variants of the *Per2* gene in mice reduce the severity of the injury after myocardial infarction because it does not only reduce inflammatory response, but also reduces apoptosis, induces cardiovascular hypertrophy, and thus preserves cardiac function [65].

Different variations of circadian rhythm genes are associated with many risk factors for cardiovascular disease. Thus, CLOCK gene variations are associated with metabolic syndrome in humans, type 2 diabetes, and some with stroke [64, 66–68], while *CRY2* and *PER2* gene variations are associated with myocardial infarction [69]. Expression of *CRY1* and *PER2* genes in fatty tissue is associated with metabolic syndrome in humans [64, 70]. Metabolic syndrome is a significant risk factor for cardiovascular disease and contributes to the common pathophysiological processes leading to the development of diabetes and cardiovascular diseases [48]. Atherosclerotic changes in blood vessels in patients with diabetes are more severe than those with normal glucose concentration [71]. It has been shown that the risk of cardiovascular disease in diabetic patients is two to three times higher than in healthy subjects [72]. Patients with diabetes usually have a higher heart rate in sleep and lower heart rate variability over the day than people without diabetes, which causes unnecessary oxygen consumption in the myocardium, with reduced nutritional blood supply. Biological and epidemiological studies suggest a direct link between lifestyle and metabolic disorders [12], although the genetic and biochemical linkage of human circadian rhythm with metabolic disorders has not been fully explored. Accordingly, the importance of the circadian rhythm in maintaining 'energy' homeostasis and metabolism is evident.

### 6.1 Cardiomyocyte circadian clock

A peripheral clock is also found in cardiomyocytes, and the internal molecular mechanism of cardiomyocytes, such as the circadian clock, might contribute to cardiovascular disease [73]. Similar to SCN, cardiomyocytes have a circadian expression of clock genes in response to serum shock or norepinephrine. Several genes are associated with intracellular metabolism or physiological activity that has a circadian expression in cardiomyocytes [74]. After development, cardiomyocytes do not replicate, although they possess a meager and permanent rate of renewal. Cardiomyocytes renew cellular structure with their new proteins and membrane lipids every few weeks [75]. The ischemic precondition is an adaptation of cardiomyocytes to hypoxia, and once the heart has suffered an ischemic insult, cardiomyocytes become more resistant to MI because of PER2 and hypoxia inducible factor (HIF)-1a [74]. Circadian genes regulate a group of genes encoding for cardiac metabolic enzymes, and it is considered that a significant role of circadian genes in the heart is to synchronize cardiomyocyte metabolic activity with the availability of nutrients in the blood (i.e., feeding time) [29]. It is known that *PER2* plays an essential role in carbohydrate metabolism during myocardial ischemia [76].

The cardiomyocyte circadian clock affects the daily variations in the heart. Studies show that the cardiomyocyte circadian clock affects myocardial contractions, the metabolism and gene expression. This clock is vital since impairment of the cardiomyocyte circadian clock might significantly alter cardiac function, cardiovascular disease pathogenesis, and treatment strategies for cardiovascular diseases (e.g., chronopharmacology) [77]. Desynchronization between different cell types (e.g., cardiomyocytes, vascular smooth muscle cells, endothelial cells) could occur within the organs (e.g. the heart) during certain physiological or pathological conditions [78]. The cardiomyocyte circadian clock allows the heart to predict circadian rhythm by extracellular stimuli, allowing rapid and temporally response [77]. The cardiomyocyte circadian clock has a crucial role in mediating the daily rhythm in myocardial metabolism and affects the cardiovascular function [79]. The cardiomyocyte circadian clock changes during illness, and this molecular mechanism might affect the etiology of cardiovascular disease [78].

## 7. Conclusions

Circadian rhythm adjusts the physiological functions of an individual on a daily basis. Daily variations of physiological parameters in the cardiovascular system maintain cardiovascular function according to the needs of different activities during the day. This information suggests that we need to know not only how, but also when to treat heart disease, and also to treat pathological changes not only symptomatically but to treat non-symptomatic but potentially harmful changes in the circadian rhythm.

Understanding the pathophysiological processes involved in the onset of myocardial infarction requires additional studies to assess the crucial elements of the circadian rhythm. In today's personalized medicine, knowledge of the circadian rhythm (i.e., the genetic background) of an individual can be significant for treatment and should be included as an essential part of the diagnostic process.

## Conflict of interest

Authors declare no conflict of interest.

## Author details

Ivana Škrlec*, Svjetlana Marić and Aleksandar Včev
Faculty of Dental Medicine and Health, J. J. Strossmayer University of Osijek, Croatia

*Address all correspondence to: iskrlec@fdmz.hr

## References

[1] Guo YF, Stein PK. Circadian rhythm in the cardiovascular system: Chronocardiology. American Heart Journal. 2003;**145**:779-786. DOI: 10.1016/S0002-8703(02)94797-6

[2] Roenneberg T, Wirz-Justice A, Merrow M. Life between clocks: Daily temporal patterns of human chronotypes. Journal of Biological Rhythms. 2003;**18**:80-90. DOI: 10.1177/0748730402239679

[3] Touitou Y, Bogdan A. Circadian and seasonal variations of physiological and biochemical determinants of acute myocardial infarction. Biological Rhythm Research. 2007;**38**:169-179. DOI: 10.1080/09291010600906075

[4] Takeda N, Maemura K. Circadian clock and vascular disease. Hypertension Research. 2010;**33**: 645-651. DOI: 10.1038/hr.2010.68

[5] Suzuki S, Ishii H, Ichimiya S, Kanashiro M, Watanabe J, Uchida Y, et al. Impact of the circadian rhythm on microvascular function in patients with ST-elevation myocardial infarction. International Journal of Cardiology. 2013;**168**:4948-4949. DOI: 10.1016/j.ijcard.2013.07.106

[6] WHO. Global Status Report on Noncommunicable Diseases 2014. Geneva. p. 2015

[7] Mendoza J. Circadian clocks: Setting time by food. Journal of Neuroendocrinology. 2007;**19**:127-137. DOI: 10.1111/j.1365-2826.2006.01510.x

[8] Chen R, Seo D-O, Bell E, von Gall C, Lee C. Strong resetting of the mammalian clock by constant light followed by constant darkness. The Journal of Neuroscience. 2008;**28**:11839-11847. DOI: 10.1523/JNEUROSCI.2191-08.2008

[9] Huang W, Ramsey KM, Marcheva B, Bass J. Circadian rhythms, sleep, and metabolism. The Journal of Clinical Investigation. 2011;**121**:2133-2141. DOI: 10.1172/JCI46043.rons

[10] Mohawk JA, Green CB, Takahashi JS. Central and peripheral circadian clocks in mammals. Annual Review of Neuroscience. 2012;**35**:445-462. DOI: 10.1146/annurev-neuro-060909-153128

[11] Gibson EM, Williams WP, Kriegsfeld LJ. Aging in the circadian system: Considerations for health, disease prevention and longevity. Experimental Gerontology. 2009;**44**: 51-56. DOI: 10.1016/j.exger.2008.05.007

[12] Dibner C, Schibler U. Circadian timing of metabolism in animal models and humans. Journal of Internal Medicine. 2015;**277**:513-527. DOI: 10.1111/joim.12347

[13] Dominguez-Rodriguez A, Abreu-Gonzalez P, Sanchez-Sanchez JJ, Kaski JC, Reiter RJ. Melatonin and circadian biology in human cardiovascular disease. Journal of Pineal Research. 2010;**49**:14-22. DOI: 10.1111/j.1600-079X.2010.00773.x

[14] Karaganis S. Non-ultradian cardiac rhythms: Circadian regulation of the heart. In: Vonend O, editor. Aspects of Pacemakers—Functions and Interactions in Cardiac and Non-Cardiac Indications. INTECH; 2011. pp. 67-88. DOI: 10.5772/845

[15] Poggiogalle E, Jamshed H, Peterson CM. Circadian regulation of glucose, lipid, and energy metabolism in humans. Metabolism. 2018;**84**:11-27. DOI: 10.1016/J.METABOL.2017.11.017

[16] Eckel-Mahan K, Sassone-Corsi P. Metabolism and the circadian clock converge. Physiological Reviews.

2013;**93**:107-135. DOI: 10.1152/physrev.00016.2012

[17] Roenneberg T, Kuehnle T, Juda M, Kantermann T, Allebrandt K, Gordijn M, et al. Epidemiology of the human circadian clock. Sleep Medicine Reviews. 2007;**11**:429-438. DOI: 10.1016/j.smrv.2007.07.005

[18] Griffett K, Burris TP. The mammalian clock and chronopharmacology. Bioorganic & Medicinal Chemistry Letters. 2013;**23**:1929-1934. DOI: 10.1016/j.bmcl.2013.02.015

[19] Roenneberg T, Merrow M. The network of time: Understanding the molecular circadian system. Current Biology. 2003;**13**:R198-R207

[20] Konopka RJ, Benzer S. Clock mutants of *Drosophila melanogaster*. PNAS. 1971;**68**:2112-2116

[21] Ohkura N, Oishi K, Fukushima N, Kasamatsu M, Atsumi G-I, Ishida N, et al. Circadian CLOCK molecules CLOCK and CRYs modulate fibrinolytic activity by regulating the PAI-1 gene expression. Journal of Thrombosis and Haemostasis. 2006;**4**:2478-2485. DOI: 10.1111/j.1538-7836.2006.02210.x

[22] Turek FW. Circadian clocks: Not your grandfather's clock. Science. 2016;**354**:992-993

[23] Antypa N, Mandelli L, Nearchou FA, Vaiopoulos C, Stefanis CN, Serretti A, et al. The 3111T/C polymorphism interacts with stressful life events to influence patterns of sleep in females. Chronobiology International. 2012;**29**:891-897. DOI: 10.3109/07420528.2012.699380

[24] Kelleher FC, Rao A, Maguire A. Circadian molecular clocks and cancer. Cancer Letters. 2014;**342**:9-18. DOI: 10.1016/j.canlet.2013.09.040

[25] Langmesser S, Tallone T, Bordon A, Rusconi S, Albrecht U. Interaction of circadian clock proteins PER2 and CRY with BMAL1 and CLOCK. BMC Molecular Biology. 2008;**9**:41. DOI: 10.1186/1471-2199-9-41

[26] Ohdo S, Koyanagi S, Matsunaga N. Chronopharmacological strategies: Intra- and inter-individual variability of molecular clock. Advanced Drug Delivery Reviews. 2010;**62**:885-897. DOI: 10.1016/j.addr.2010.04.005

[27] Partch CL, Green CB, Takahashi JS. Molecular architecture of the mammalian circadian clock. Trends in Cell Biology. 2014;**24**:90-99. DOI: 10.1016/j.tcb.2013.07.002

[28] Takeda N, Maemura K. Cardiovascular disease, chronopharmacotherapy, and the molecular clock. Advanced Drug Delivery Reviews. 2010;**62**:956-966. DOI: 10.1016/j.addr.2010.04.011

[29] Virag JAI, Lust RM. Circadian influences on myocardial infarction. Frontiers in Physiology. 2014;**5**:422. DOI: 10.3389/fphys.2014.00422

[30] Kumar J, P Challet E, Kalsbeek A. Circadian rhythms in glucose and lipid metabolism in nocturnal and diurnal mammals. Molecular and Cellular Endocrinology. 2015;**418**:74-88. DOI: 10.1016/j.mce.2015.01.024

[31] Leu H-B, Chung C-M, Lin S-J, Chiang K-M, Yang H-C, Ho H-Y, et al. Association of circadian genes with diurnal blood pressure changes and non-dipper essential hypertension: A genetic association with young-onset hypertension. Hypertension Research. 2015;**38**:155-162. DOI: 10.1038/hr.2014.152

[32] Gómez-Abellán P, Madrid JA, Ordovás JM, Garaulet M. Chronobiological aspects of obesity and metabolic syndrome. Endocrinología

y Nutrición. 2012;**59**:50-61. DOI: 10.1016/j.endoen.2011.08.002

[33] Gale JE, Cox HI, Qian J, Block GD, Colwell CS, Matveyenko AV. Disruption of circadian rhythms accelerates development of diabetes through pancreatic beta-cell loss and dysfunction. Journal of Biological Rhythms. 2011;**26**:423-433. DOI: 10.1177/0748730411416341

[34] Kovanen L, Saarikoski ST, Haukka J, Pirkola S, Aromaa A, Lönnqvist J, et al. Circadian clock gene polymorphisms in alcohol use disorders and alcohol consumption. Alcohol and Alcoholism. 2010;**45**:303-311. DOI: 10.1093/alcalc/agq035

[35] Pedrazzoli M, Secolin R, Esteves LOB, Pereira DS, Koike BDV, Louzada FM, et al. Interactions of polymorphisms in different clock genes associated with circadian phenotypes in humans. Genetics and Molecular Biology. 2010;**33**:627-632. DOI: 10.1590/S1415-47572010005000092

[36] Kovanen L, Donner K, Kaunisto M, Partonen T. CRY1, CRY2 and PRKCDBP genetic variants in metabolic syndrome. Hypertension Research. 2015;**38**:186-192. DOI: 10.1038/hr.2014.157

[37] Dashti HS, Smith CE, Lee Y-C, Parnell LD, Lai C-Q, Arnett DK, et al. CRY1 circadian gene variant interacts with carbohydrate intake for insulin resistance in two independent populations: Mediterranean and North American. Chronobiology International. 2014;**31**:660-667. DOI: 10.3109/07420528.2014.886587

[38] Young MW, Kay SA. Time zones: A comparative genetics of circadian clocks. Nature Reviews. Genetics. 2001;**2**:702-715. DOI: 10.1038/35088576

[39] Mongrain V, Cermakian N. Clock genes in health and diseases. Journal of Applied Biomedicine. 2009;**7**:15-33

[40] Cornelissen G. Metabolic syndrome, adiponectin, sleep, and the circadian system. eBioMedicine. 2018;**33**:20-21. DOI: 10.1016/J.EBIOM.2018.06.013

[41] Crnko S, Cour M, Van Laake LW, Lecour S. Vasculature on the clock: Circadian rhythm and vascular dysfunction. Vascular Pharmacology. 2018;**108**:1-7. DOI: 10.1016/J.VPH.2018.05.003

[42] WHO. Noncommunicable Diseases Progress Monitor 2017. Geneva; 2017. p. 231

[43] Kralj V, Brkić BI. Mortalitet i morbiditet od kardiovaskularnih bolesti. Cardiologia Croatica. 2013;**8**:373-378

[44] Tengattini S, Reiter RJ, Tan D-X, Terron MP, Rodella LF, Rezzani R. Cardiovascular diseases: Protective effects of melatonin. Journal of Pineal Research. 2008;**44**:16-25. DOI: 10.1111/j.1600-079X.2007.00518.x

[45] Matura LA. Gender and circadian effects of myocardial infarctions. Clinical Nursing Research. 2010;**19**:55-70. DOI: 10.1177/1054773809354371

[46] Knutson KL. Sleep duration and cardiometabolic risk: A review of the epidemiologic evidence. Best Practice & Research. Clinical Endocrinology & Metabolism. 2010;**24**:731-743. DOI: 10.1016/j.beem.2010.07.001

[47] Morgan TM, Xiao L, Lyons P, Kassebaum B, Krumholz HM, Spertus JA. Investigation of 89 candidate gene variants for effects on all-cause mortality following acute coronary syndrome. BMC Medical Genetics. 2008;**9**:66. DOI: 10.1186/1471-2350-9-66

[48] Prasai MJ, George JT, Scott EM. Molecular clocks, type 2 diabetes and cardiovascular disease. Diabetes and Vascular Disease Research. 2008;**5**:89-95. DOI: 10.3132/dvdr.2008.015

[49] Marcheva B, Ramsey KM, Buhr ED, Kobayashi Y, Su H, Ko CH, et al. Disruption of the CLOCK components CLOCK and BMAL1 leads to hypoinsulinaemia and diabetes. Nature. 2010;**466**:627-631. DOI: 10.1038/nature09253

[50] Thygesen K, Alpert JS, White HD. Universal definition of myocardial infarction. European Heart Journal. 2007;**28**:2525-2538. DOI: 10.1093/eurheartj/ehm355

[51] Domínguez-Rodríguez A, Abreu-González P, García MJ, Sanchez J, Marrero F, de Armas-Trujillo D. Decreased nocturnal melatonin levels during acute myocardial infarction. Journal of Pineal Research. 2002;**33**:248-252

[52] Klinkenberg LJJ, van Dijk J-W, Tan FES, van Loon LJC, van Dieijen-Visser MP, Meex SJR. Circulating cardiac troponin T exhibits a diurnal rhythm. Journal of the American College of Cardiology. 2014;**63**:1788-1795. DOI: 10.1016/j.jacc.2014.01.040

[53] Thygesen K, Alpert JS, Jaffe AS, Simoons ML, Chaitman BR, White HD. Third universal definition of myocardial infarction. Nature Reviews. Cardiology. 2012;**9**:620-633. DOI: 10.1038/nrcardio.2012.122

[54] Saaby L, Poulsen TS, Hosbond S, Larsen TB, Pyndt Diederichsen AC, Hallas J, et al. Classification of myocardial infarction: Frequency and features of type 2 myocardial infarction. The American Journal of Medicine. 2013;**126**:789-797. DOI: 10.1016/j.amjmed.2013.02.029

[55] Alpert JS, Thygesen KA, White HD, Jaffe AS. Diagnostic and therapeutic implications of type 2 myocardial infarction: Review and commentary. The American Journal of Medicine. 2014;**127**:105-108. DOI: 10.1016/j.amjmed.2013.09.031

[56] Erdmann J, Linsel-Nitschke P, Schunkert H. Genetic causes of myocardial infarction: New insights from genome-wide association studies. Deutsches Ärzteblatt International. 2010;**107**:694-699. DOI: 10.3238/arztebl.2010.0694

[57] Kanth R, Ittaman S, Rezkalla S. Circadian patterns of ST elevation myocardial infarction in the new millennium. Clinical Medicine & Research. 2013;**11**:66-72. DOI: 10.3121/cmr.2013.1120

[58] Chong NW, Codd V, Chan D, Samani NJ. Circadian clock genes cause activation of the human PAI-1 gene promoter with 4G/5G allelic preference. FEBS Letters. 2006;**580**:4469-4472. DOI: 10.1016/j.febslet.2006.07.014

[59] Tsimakouridze E, Alibhai F, Martino T. Therapeutic applications of circadian rhythms for the cardiovascular system. Frontiers in Pharmacology. 2015;**6**:1-10. DOI: 10.3389/fphar.2015.00077

[60] Chowta K, Prijith P, Chowta M, Prabhu M. Circadian pattern in the onset of acute myocardial infarction. Indian Academy of Clinical Medicine Journal. 2006;7:206-210

[61] Sheikh M, Murshad N, Majid A, Abid A, Malik S, Mallick N. Infuence of circadian variations on onset and in-hospital outcome of first acute myocardial infarction. Pakistan Heart Journal. 2010;**43**:31-38

[62] Chan C-M, Chen W-L, Kuo H-Y, Huang C-C, Shen Y-S, Choy C-S, et al. Circadian variation of acute myocardial infarction in young people. The American Journal of Emergency Medicine. 2012;**30**:1461-1465. DOI: 10.1016/j.ajem.2011.11.019

[63] López F, Lee KW, Marín F, Roldán V, Sogorb F, Caturla J, et al. Are there ethnic differences in the circadian variation in onset of acute myocardial

infarction? A comparison of 3 ethnic groups in Birmingham, UK and Alicante, Spain. International Journal of Cardiology. 2005;**100**:151-154. DOI: 10.1016/j.ijcard.2004.12.002

[64] Scott EM. Circadian clocks, obesity and cardiometabolic function. Diabetes, Obesity and Metabolism. 2015;**17**:84-89. DOI: 10.1111/dom.12518

[65] Virag JAI, Dries JL, Easton PR, Friesland AM, Deantonio JH, Chintalgattu V, et al. Attenuation of myocardial injury in mice with functional deletion of the circadian rhythm gene mPer2. American Journal of Physiology-Heart and Circulatory Physiology. 2010;**198**:H1088-H1095

[66] Scott EM, Carter AM, Grant PJ. Association between polymorphisms in the clock gene, obesity and the metabolic syndrome in man. International Journal of Obesity. 2008;**32**:658-662. DOI: 10.1038/sj.ijo.0803778

[67] Corella D, Asensio EM, Coltell O, Sorlí JV, Estruch R, Martínez-González MÁ, et al. CLOCK gene variation is associated with incidence of type-2 diabetes and cardiovascular diseases in type-2 diabetic subjects: Dietary modulation in the PREDIMED randomized trial. Cardiovascular Diabetology. 2016;**15**:4. DOI: 10.1186/s12933-015-0327-8

[68] Škrlec I. Varijabilnost gena cirkadijalnog ritma u osoba s infarktom miokarda [thesis]. Osijek: Faculty of Medicine; 2018

[69] Škrlec I, Milić J, Heffer M, Peterlin B, Wagner J. Genetic variations in circadian rhythm genes and susceptibility for myocardial infarction. Genetics and Molecular Biology. 2018;**41**:403-409. DOI: 10.1590/1678-4685-gmb-2017-0147

[70] Gómez-Abellán P, Hernández-Morante JJ, Luján JA, Madrid JA, Garaulet M. Clock genes are implicated in the human metabolic syndrome. International Journal of Obesity. 2008;**32**:121-128. DOI: 10.1038/sj.ijo.0803689

[71] Paneni F, Beckman JA, Creager MA, Cosentino F. Diabetes and vascular disease: Pathophysiology, clinical consequences, and medical therapy: Part I. European Heart Journal. 2013;**34**:2436-2443. DOI: 10.1093/eurheartj/eht149

[72] Martín-Timón I, Sevillano-Collantes C, Segura-Galindo A, Del Cañizo-Gómez FJ. Type 2 diabetes and cardiovascular disease: Have all risk factors the same strength? World Journal of Diabetes. 2014;**5**:444-470. DOI: 10.4239/wjd.v5.i4.444

[73] Suárez-Barrientos A, López-Romero P, Vivas D, Castro-Ferreira F, Núñez-Gil I, Franco E, et al. Circadian variations of infarct size in acute myocardial infarction. Heart. 2011;**97**:970-976. DOI: 10.1136/hrt.2010.212621

[74] Takeda N, Maemura K. The role of clock genes and circadian rhythm in the development of cardiovascular diseases. Cellular and Molecular Life Sciences. 2015;**72**:3225-3234. DOI: 10.1007/s00018-015-1923-1

[75] Martino TA, Sole MJ. Molecular time: An often overlooked dimension to cardiovascular disease. Circulation Research. 2009;**105**:1047-1061. DOI: 10.1161/CIRCRESAHA.109.206201

[76] Bonney S, Kominsky D, Brodsky K, Eltzschig H, Walker L, Eckle T. Cardiac Per2 functions as novel link between fatty acid metabolism and myocardial inflammation during ischemia and reperfusion injury of the heart. PLoS One. 2013;**8**:e71493. DOI: 10.1371/journal.pone.0071493

[77] Bray MS, Shaw CA, Moore MWS, Garcia RAP, Zanquetta MM, Durgan DJ, et al. Disruption of the circadian clock within the cardiomyocyte influences myocardial contractile function, metabolism, and gene expression. American Journal of Physiology-Heart and Circulatory Physiology. 2008;**294**:H1036-H1047. DOI: 10.1152/ajpheart.01291.2007

[78] Durgan DJ, Young ME. The cardiomyocyte circadian clock: Emerging roles in health and disease. Circulation Research. 2010;**106**:647-658. DOI: 10.1161/CIRCRESAHA.109.209957

[79] Chatham JC, Young ME. Regulation of myocardial metabolism by the cardiomyocyte circadian clock. Journal of Molecular and Cellular Cardiology. 2013;**55**:139-146. DOI: 10.1016/J.YJMCC.2012.06.016

Section 2

# Myocardial Genetics

Chapter 4

# Current Pathophysiological and Genetic Aspects of Dilated Cardiomyopathy

*Deborah P. Schild, Sascha I. Ricciardi, Jens G. Hellige, Rolf Vogel and Nisha Arenja*

## Abstract

Dilated cardiomyopathy is the most common form of cardiomyopathy and the second leading cause of left ventricular dysfunction with highly variable clinical presentation and prognosis. The clinical courses vary and are strongly heterogeneous, ranging from asymptomatic patients to those suffering from intractable heart failure or sudden cardiac death due to arrhythmias. Previous studies have reported a 10 years cardiovascular mortality up to 40% in developed countries, due to advanced heart failure or sudden cardiac death. However, the prognosis of dilated cardiomyopathy patients is variable and depends on multiple risk factors. This chapter provides a review of dilated cardiomyopathy with specific focus on the pathophysiological aspects and genetic etiology of the disease.

**Keywords:** dilated cardiomyopathy, pathophysiology, etiology, diagnostics, therapy

## 1. Introduction

Dilated cardiomyopathy (DCM) is one of the most common cardiomyopathies causing heart failure (HF) worldwide. Although it is less common than coronary artery disease (CAD), it affects mainly young adults and presents the most frequent reason for cardiac transplantation in young age [1, 2]. According to the European Society of Cardiology (ESC), the current definition of DCM includes the presence of a dilated and poorly functioning left ventricle or of both ventricles [3]. A heterogeneous group of myocardial and systemic conditions may cause left ventricular dilatation in combination with dysfunction. In fact, identifying the etiology of DCM can be very challenging, which often leads to the common terminology of idiopathic dilated cardiomyopathy (IDC). Furthermore, DCM has a highly variable clinical presentation. While signs and symptoms of HF are most common, some patients are incidentally, for instance, by diagnosing cardiomegaly in chest X-ray. Other symptoms include arrhythmias, conduction disturbances, thromboembolic complications, or sudden cardiac death (SCD). In the last decades, major advances have been made in the understanding of molecular and genetic issues, as well as in the pathophysiology and clinical assessment of cardiomyopathies. Especially, understanding the genetic basis of DCM has improved considerably with the availability of genetic analysis. In addition, other important diagnostic approaches, particularly imaging methods are more widely available. This allows early diagnosis and the initiation of adequate therapy, which already has led to an improvement of the prognosis in the last years. Data have shown that approximately 25% of DCM patients with recent onset of HF (<6 months) have ameliorated in symptoms or even have complete cardiac function recovery [4, 5]. However, the overall prognosis in patients with symptomatic HF and DCM is still poor. In order to further improve the prognosis of our patients, it is important to regularly gather the knowledge about the current state of DCM and adapt the appropriate diagnostic workups. Therefore, this chapter provides the reader with a comprehensive overview of the current state of DCM from definition over etiology including the genetics aspects to management for cardiovascular specialists.

## 2. Dilated cardiomyopathy: a frequent cardiac disease

### 2.1 Definition

In 1980, the World Health Organization (WHO) defined cardiomyopathies as "heart muscle diseases of unknown cause" [6]. The definition was established to distinguish cardiomyopathies from cardiac diseases with known entities such as hypertension, ischemic, or valvular heart disease. About 15 years later, the WHO/ International Society and Federation of Cardiology (ISFC) Task Force classified cardiomyopathies according to anatomy and physiology into dilated cardiomyopathy (DCM), hypertrophic cardiomyopathy (HCM), restrictive cardiomyopathy (RCM), arrhythmogenic right ventricular cardiomyopathy/dysplasia (ARVC/D) and unclassified cardiomyopathies. The definitions and classifications of cardiomyopathies changed over the years. The American Heart Association (AHA) presented a new scheme in 2006 that combined genetic and clinical criteria [7]. In contrast to that, the ESC defined in 2008 cardiomyopathies in a more clinically oriented classification system according to the WHO scheme as myocardial disorders with structurally and functionally abnormities of the heart muscle in the absence of coronary artery disease, hypertension, valvular disease, or congenital heart disease [3]. As mentioned above, right ventricular dilatation and dysfunction may be present but are not necessary for the diagnosis. Further, DCM is classified into familial/genetic and nonfamilial/nongenetic forms [3]. Recently, a revised definition of DCM was presented by the ESC working group on myocardial and pericardial diseases [8]. This position paper did not modify the above-mentioned definition, it rather added the important value of diverse etiologies and clinical manifestations with an introduction of a novel concept of a continuous phenotypic DCM spectrum, ranging from the subclinical mutation carriers to fully expressed DCM phenotypes.

### 2.2 Prevalence

The prevalence of DCM in the general population is unknown. The reported numbers considerably vary due to inhomogeneous study methodologies, which are mainly related to inconsistent definitions and classifications of DCM. In addition, the prevalence of DCM varies according to geographic and ethnic differences. One of the first reports was derived from an epidemiological study conducted in Olmsted County, Minnesota, from 1975 to 1984. For the diagnosis of DCM, the authors implemented echocardiography, angiography, and autopsy cases [9]. They presented a prevalence of 36.5/100,000 individuals or 1 in 2700 with a male to female ratio of 3:4 in a European-American population. A much higher prevalence with 1:250 was reported recently by a study from Hershberger et al. The authors estimated the DCM prevalence based on the known ratio of idiopathic DCM to

HCM of ≈2:1. In addition, clinical data of HF patients and left ventricular dysfunction were used as a surrogate for DCM [10]. In Western countries, 25–40% of DCM patients have been described with evidence of familial DCM with predominantly autosomal dominant inheritance [4, 11–13]. In general, epidemiologic studies have stated a rate of 20 up to >50% of familial DCM in patients, who were initially diagnosed with IDC [9, 11, 14–18].

## 2.3 Clinical presentation

The first presentation of patients with DCM is often characterized by signs and symptoms of HF, such as dyspnea, ankle swelling, fatigue, elevated jugular venous pressure, pulmonary rales, and peripheral edema (**Table 1**). These result from reduced cardiac function with low output and/or elevated intracardiac pressures. Other clinical manifestations include chest pain caused by reduced coronary blood flow or congestion, palpitations, and syncope or sudden cardiac death (SCD). Arrhythmia results from multifactorial reasons, which are present in DCM and include structural changes with myocardial fibrosis and left ventricular dilation as well as electrophysiological changes [19]. The risk of SCD is highly heterogeneous and depends on etiologies and risk factors [20]. Some genetic constellations may be associated with arrhythmias out of proportion to the degree of left ventricular dysfunction (e.g., pathogenic variants in DES, LMNA, and SCN5A) [21]. This is described later in this chapter (see Sections 2.7.3 and 2.8). Furthermore, patients might present with pulmonary and systemic thromboembolism [22]. Possible clinical findings are summarized in **Table 1**.

| | Cardiac | Pulmonary | Gastrointestinal/ urogenital | Other |
|---|---|---|---|---|
| Symptoms | Chest pain<br>Palpitations<br>Syncope | Dyspnea<br>Wheeze<br>Blood-tinged sputum<br>Cough | Reduced appetite<br>Epigastral pain<br>Bloating<br>Obstipation<br>Diarrhea<br>Swollen abdomen<br>Nycturia<br>Reduced libido<br>Erectile dysfunction | Dizziness<br>Lightheadness<br>Concentration disturbances<br>Fatigue<br>Fainting<br>Sweating<br>Leg swelling<br>Symptoms of multisystem disease<br>Skin alterations<br>Visual and hearing impairment<br>Gait disturbance |
| Clinical signs | Hypotonia<br>Tachycardia<br>Pulsus alternans<br>Arrhythmia<br>Third heart sound<br>Loud 2nd heart sound<br>Displaced apex beat<br>Elevated jugular venous pressure<br>Eedema | Tachycardia<br>Tachypnoea<br>Low oxygen saturation<br>Hemoptysis<br>Rales<br>Obstructive lung auscultation<br>Diminished lung sounds due to pleural effusions<br>Pulmonary edema | Hepatomegaly<br>Ascites<br>Jaundice in terminal liver failure<br>Cachexia | Intellectual disability<br>Deafness<br>Myotonia<br>Hyperpigmentation<br>Palmoplantar keratoderma<br>Woolly hair<br>Dysmorphic appearance<br>Polyneuropathic symptoms<br>Carpal tunnel syndrome |

**Table 1.**
*Clinical findings in dilated cardiomyopathy.*

## 2.4 Pathophysiological aspects and etiology

As a consequence of the definition, the etiology of left ventricular dilatation and dysfunction is heterogeneous. In developed countries, CAD is the most common cause of left ventricular dilatation and dysfunction, and responsible for approximately 50–70% of HF patients. Therefore, potentially reversible myocardial ischemia must always be excluded for the diagnosis of DCM. The following section describes in detail the possible causes of the DCM (**Figure 1**). However, the current literature underscores that the cause of DCM remains unknown, that is, IDC, in half of the patients [23].

### *2.4.1 Non-genetic causes of DCM*

#### *2.4.1.1 Inflammatory cardiomyopathy*

DCM can occur after a cardiac infection or inflammation as an early (e.g. giant-cell myocarditis) or late stage disease. Typically, the active or fulminant myocarditis appears with preserved left ventricular size, while in contrast inflammatory DCM is defined as the presence of chronic inflammatory cells in association with left ventricular dilatation and reduced fraction [3]. The inflammatory myocarditis can result from an infection or may be mediated by autoimmune mechanisms. The infectious myocarditis is commonly caused by viral pathogens as an acute or chronic disease [24]. In the developed countries until the 1990s, the most frequently reported viruses were adenoviruses and enteroviruses. Recently, parvovirus B12 and human herpes virus-6 are increasingly reported causing DCM [25]. In the acute phase, the virus replicates actively within the myocardium. This leads to dysfunction of cardiomyocytes and endothelial cells, and thus triggering the immune response [23]. Commonly, the innate immune system clears the viral load whereas insufficient immune response results in viral persistence and progressive myocyte destruction [25]. The secondary effect is triggered by primed T-cells. In addition, some host myocardial cellular antigens may share epitopic similarities with viral antigens and induce an autoimmune response with further destruction of cardiomyocytes [23].

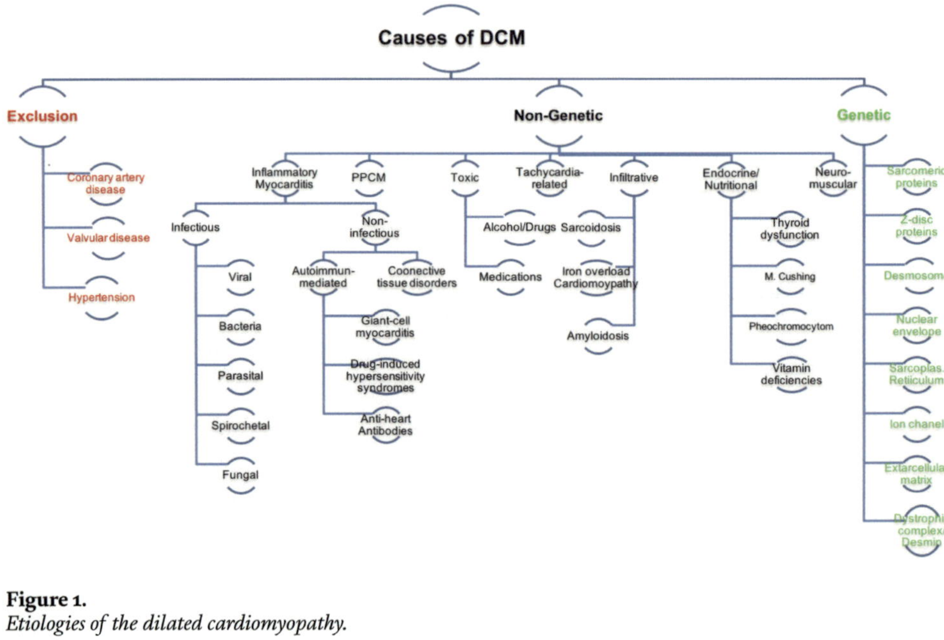


**Figure 1.**
*Etiologies of the dilated cardiomyopathy.*

Another important viral-related form of DCM is HIV syndrome. DCM in HIV patients is called HIV-associated cardiomyopathy. Autopsies demonstrated histological evidence of myocarditis in around 50% of patients, who died of AIDS-related illness [26]. Bacterial infections such as brucellosis, diphtheria, psittacosis, and typhoid fever are also known to cause (peri-) myocarditis [27–30]. In addition, E. coli bacteraemia have been described to induce myocarditis [31]. Spirochaetal myocarditis may be encountered in the setting of the Lyme disease (Borrelia burgdorferi), the Weil disease (Leptospirosis), and syphilis (Treponema pallidum) [32]. In endemic areas, the protozoan parasite Trypanosoma cruzi is a typical cause of DCM due to acute cardiac infection (perimyocarditis), as well as chronic myocardial fibrosis leading to DCM [33]. There are several proposed mechanisms leading to DCM in autoimmune disorders. These include immune-mediated myocarditis, progressive fibrosis, apoptosis with resultant restrictive and dilated phenotypes, and progressive atherosclerosis with subsequent ischemic cardiomyopathy [26]. Other causes for a non-infectious myocarditis are: Kawasaki disease in children with coronary vasculitis and systemic lupus erythematosus, which can affect the myocardium without involvement of the pericardium. In rare cases, connective tissue diseases such as scleroderma, rheumatoid arthritis, and polyarteritis nodosa may lead to DCM [26]. The non-infectious etiologies of myocarditis include drug-induced hypersensitivity and hypereosinophilic syndromes, as well as giant-cell myocarditis, which is one of the most aggressive non-infectious autoimmune disorders with rapid and devastating outcome if not treated appropriately [24, 26].

#### *2.4.1.2 Peripartum cardiomyopathy*

Peripartum cardiomyopathy (PPCM) affects predisposed teenagers and older women during the last month of pregnancy or within 5 months of delivery with typical signs and symptoms of HF [34, 35]. Suspected etiological factors include inflammatory myocarditis, autoimmunity caused by chimerism of hematopoietic lineage cells from the fetus, hemodynamic stress during pregnancy, and toxicity caused by an abnormal cleavage product of prolactin [3, 36]. Furthermore, genetic predisposition seems to be important [37].

#### *2.4.1.3 Toxic cardiomyopathies*

A number of chemical compounds are responsible for DCM. In western and developing countries, alcoholic cardiomyopathy (ACM) represents one of the most common forms of secondary cardiomyopathies resembling IDC with an estimated prevalence of 23–40% [24, 38]. More than women, men are affected by ACM and the occurrence correlates with a daily level and the duration of alcohol consumption [39]. However, the prevalence of ACM is variable and the mean daily amount of alcohol consumption, duration of regular intake, and patients' individual characteristics, including genetic susceptibility, are all related to the development of a respective cardiomyopathy [26]. Alcohol may result in both acute and chronic depression of myocardial contractility. Street drugs such as cocaine and methamphetamines are potent sympathomimetic drugs that induce inotropic and chronotropic effects. Mechanisms of cardiac toxicity include myocardial ischemia from increased oxygen consumption, prothrombotic effects, coronary vasospasms, and acceleration of coronary atherosclerosis [24]. Anthracycline-based chemotherapeutic agents are known to induce cardiac dysfunction. Acute or subacute injury can occur immediately after treatment with transient arrhythmias, pericarditis, and myocarditis [38]. The time course of chronic development of HF varies from an early onset (<1 year) to late onset (>1 year) or chronic progressive cardiomyopathy, which can occur 10–30 years after exposure. Both chronic forms tend to be irreversible, are dosage dependent and are associated with ultrastructural changes in the cardiac myocytes [40]. Trastuzumab, a monoclonal antibody directed against the human epidermal growth factor receptor 2 (HER2), is wildly used and very effective for the treatment of HER2-positive breast cancer. HER2 receptors are also localized on the cardiomyocyte. The inhibition of the Her2:Her4 signaling process in the myocardium is principally responsible for the cardiotoxicity [26]. In addition, a number of other, non-chemotherapeutical medications are associated with DCM, such as cyclophosphamide, phenothiazines, antidepressant drugs, carbon monoxide, lead, lithium, pseudoephedrine, ephedrine, cobalt, anabolic steroids, hydroxychloroquine, clozapine, and catecholamines [38, 41]. Possible causes of toxic cardiomyopathy are summarized in **Figure 2**.

#### *2.4.1.4 Arrhythmia-induced DCM*

Tachycardia-induced cardiomyopathy was described more than 100 years ago by Gossage et al. as a reversible form of systolic dysfunction caused by long-lasting supraventricular or ventricular arrhythmias [42]. Ongoing rapid atrial or ventricular pacing may result in systemic changes by neurohormonal activation, characterized by reduction in serum sodium, activation of the renin-angiotensin system, and an increase of plasma atrial natriuretic peptide, aldosterone, and norepinephrine. Abnormal myocardial and cellular remodeling occurs, which may result in DCM. Furthermore, epinephrine can also lead to abnormal myocardial and cellular remodeling, which further result in biventricular dilatation, decreased contractility, and elevation of left and/or biventricular filling pressure [26].

#### *2.4.1.5 Infiltrative diseases*

Several, systemic diseases may infiltrate the myocardium and result in DCM. Sarcoidosis, iron overload, and amyloidosis represent the most common clinical entities. Sarcoidosis is a multisystem inflammatory disease of unknown origin characterized by non-caseating granulomas in multiple organs. Sarcoidosis can progress to a fibrotic stage leading to DCM [26]. In the setting of iron overload, such as hereditary hematochromatosis, high blood volume, or parenteral iron infusions,

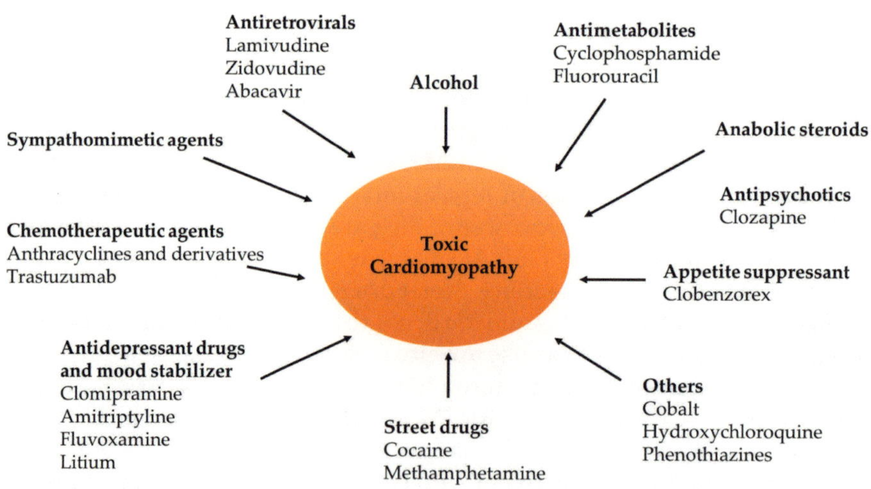


**Figure 2.**
*Reasons for toxic cardiomyopathies.*

DCM may occur due to iron-induced reactive oxygen species with cellular oxidative stress and fibrosis [43]. Cardiac amyloidosis is the most common cause of infiltrative cardiomyopathy with poor prognosis. Amyloid is an extracellular tissue deposition of misfolded amyloid protein-fibrils [44]. Cardiac amyloidosis usually presents as a cardiomyopathy with restrictive pathophysiology and can progress to severe cardiac dysfunction and to DCM in very advanced stages [26].

#### *2.4.1.6 Endocrine/metabolic disorders*

Endocrinologic disorders rarely lead to the phenotype of DCM. Especially thyroid hormones have a significant impact on cardiac function and structure via regulation and expression of key structural and regulatory genes like myosin heavy chain and phospholamban. Therefore, excess or deficiency of triiodothyronine (T3) may lead to DCM in a late stage [45]. Growth hormone disorders, pheochromocytoma, and Cushing's disease are also very rare causes of DCM [26, 46]. Furthermore, the literature names nutritional deficiencies of thiamine (beriberi disease), selenium (Keshan disease), and L-carnitine being responsible for DCM [47, 48].

#### *2.4.1.7 Neuromuscular disorders*

Neuromuscular disease like Duchenne's muscular dystrophy, Becker muscular dystrophy, and Emery-Dreifuss muscular dystrophy can affect the heart and induce DCM. Patients with DCM and muscular dystrophy commonly show X-linked mutations or autosomal recessive inheritance [24]. Further information is summarized in the following section on genetic causes of DCM.

### *2.4.2 Genetic causes of DCM*

In up to 30% of the cases, a gene mutation may be identified as the main cause of DCM [49]. Thanks to advances in next-generation sequencing technologies more than 40 genes have already been identified causing DCM [50]. Most commonly, familial DCM is inherited as an autosomal dominant pattern. Autosomal recessive, X-linked, and mitochondrial inheritance patterns are less common [24]. Most of the genes involved in the development of DCM encode structural elements of the cardiomyocytes. Mutations in genes encoding sarcomeric, cytoskeletal, desmosomal, nuclear membrane, mitochondrial, and RNA-binding proteins have all been linked to DCM [51]. Interestingly, several of the gene mutations linked to autosomal dominant DCM encode the same contractile proteins that are also responsible for the development of HCM [38]. As well, other affected genes are described in ARVC and left ventricular non-compaction cardiomyopathy (NCCM). In the following, we will describe the most investigated gene mutations and their consequences on the cardiomyocyte functioning.

#### *2.4.2.1 Sarcomere protein location: force generation and transmission*

The sarcomere is the contracting unit of the myocyte. The thin filaments of the sarcomere emanate from the Z-disc. They consist of filamentous α-actin (gene name ACTC 1) and calcium-sensitive troponin-tropomyosin regulatory apparatus (encoded by TPM1), which includes the three troponin subunits (encoded by TNNT2, TNNC1, and TNNI3) [52, 53]. The thick filament core is formed by the β-myosin heavy chain (encoded by MYH7), the molecular motor of the thick filament, and the myosin-binding protein C (β-MYBPC3) [52, 53]. Titin (encoded by TTN), which is the largest human protein, spans the half length of the sarcomere, where it acts as a stretch sensor and myofibril stabilizer. It limits sarcomere stretch in early diastole and restores resting sarcomere length after contraction [52, 53]. Titin (TTN) mutations are the most prevalent genetic cause of idiopathic DCM (15–20%). In fact, DCM patients with TTN mutations have a worse outcome due to a higher arrhythmic risk and progressive functional deficits [54]. Mutations in human genes encoding protein components of the sarcomere cause either HCM or DCM. Deficits of force production and transmission are the two main mechanisms that lead to DCM due to sarcomere mutations [55]. Mutations of genes encoding myosin proteins (MYH 6, MYH7, and MYBPC3), actin proteins (ACTC 1 and ACTC 2), and tropomyosin protein (TPM 1) result in alterations of coupling-uncoupling mechanisms of actin to myosin [50]. Specifically, TPM1 mutations are associated with destabilization of actin interactions and compromise force transmission to neighboring sarcomeres. ACTC mutations impair the binding of actin to the Z-disc compromising force propagation [55]. Impaired contractile force may also occur from troponin mutations. Because troponin molecules modulate calcium-stimulated actomyosin ATPase activity, the mutation causes inefficient ATP hydrolysis and decrease contractile strength [55].

#### *2.4.2.2 Cytoskeleton protein location: force transmission and structural integrity*

The Z-disc is an electron-dense structure, in which titin and the thin filaments anchor. Critical components include α-actinin, which aligns actin and titin from neighboring sarcomeres and interacts with muscle LIM protein (MLP encoded by CSRP3). Telethonin (encoded by TCAP) is another Z-disc component interacting with titin and MLP to support overall sarcomere function. In addition, Cipher/Z-band alternatively spliced PDZ-motif protein (Cipher/ZASP encoded by LDB3), which interacts with α-actinin-2 through a PDZ domain, an abundant protein interaction modules that recognize short amino acid motifs of the C-termini of target proteins, and couples to protein kinase C (PKC)-mediated signaling via its LIM domains [55, 56]. Gene mutations of multiple Z-disc proteins like MLP, cardiac ankyrin repeat protein (CARP), myopalladin, α-actinin 2, TCAP, and nexilin may result in DCM [52]. Cipher/ZASP mutations have been associated to isolated left ventricular dilatation or DCM with NCCM phenotype [50]. Metavinculin (encoded by VCL) attaches the thin filaments to the plasma membrane and plays a key role in force transmission. Gene mutations in metavinculin cause DCM by disruption of disc structure and actin-filament organization [55]. The costamere, a rib-like structure of the cytoplasmatic and transmembrane proteins, interconnects the cytoskeleton to the plasma membrane and the extracellular matrix. Dystrophin and its associated proteins, sacroglycans and dystroglycan, enrich at the costamere and protect against contraction-induced injury [52]. The integrity of the dystrophin complex is critical for mechano-transduction and loss of function mutations trigger instability of the plasma membrane and myofiber loss. This mechanism leads to Duchenne and Becker muscular dystrophy [57]. Desmin, another intermediate filament in cardiomyocytes, forms a 3D scaffold that extends across the entire diameter of the cardiomyocyte, surrounds the Z-discs and interlinks them together and integrates the contractile apparatus with the sarcolemma and the nucleus. Desmin helps to sense mechanical stretch and transduces downstream signals from extracellular to the nucleus. In addition, desmin plays a crucial role during myogenesis. Inhibition of desmin expression blocks myoblast fusion and myotube formation [58]. Mutations in the desmin genes are associated with an autosomal dominant skeletal myopathy, cardiac conduction block, and DCM [59]. Prevalence of desmin mutations in familial DCM have been reported in 1–2% [60].

#### *2.4.2.3 Desmosomes: cell-cell adhesion and intracellular signaling/mechano-signaling*

Desmosomes are organized cell membrane structures that provide functional and structural contact between adjacent cells. Mutations in protein components of desmosomes like plakoglobin, desmoplakin, and plakophilin-2 can cause syndromic and non-syndromic ARVC as well as DCM due to disruption of intercellular junction [55, 61].

#### *2.4.2.4 Sarcoplasmic reticulum: calcium homeostasis*

Calcium enters the myocyte through voltage-gated L-type $Ca^{2+}$-channels. This triggers the release of calcium from the sarcoplasmic reticulum (SR) via the ryanodine receptor 2 (RyR2). At low intracellular calcium concentrations, troponin I and actin interactions block actomyosin ATPase activity. With increasing intracellular concentration, calcium binds to troponin C, which releases troponin I inhibition and stimulates contraction. Calcium dissociates from troponin C in cardiac relaxation. Calcium concentration decreases by calcium reuptake in the SR through the phospholamban-regulated cardiac sarcoplasmic reticulum $CA^{2+}$-ATPase (SERCA2a) [55]. Mutations of phospholamban precipitate DCM by altering calcium homeostasis [54]. Specific phospholamban mutation R14del is associated with high risk of malignant ventricular arrhythmias and end-stage HF. Further, it is described in a phenotype of ARVC [62].

#### *2.4.2.5 Nuclear envelope: maintain structural organization*

The nuclear membrane protein complex contains emerin and lamin A/C (LMNA) [52, 55]. These two lamina proteins and nesprin-1 are part of the LINC complex that links the nucleus to the cytoplasm. Stress signals in the cytoplasm are hypothesized to act with the LINC complex, affecting gene expression in the nucleus. The LINC complex is crucial for an appropriate transcriptional response of the cell to mechanical stress [52]. Defects in emerin proteins can induce X-linked Emery-Dreifuss muscular dystrophy, joint contractures, conduction system disease, and DCM. Dominant lamin A/C (encoded by LMNA) mutations exhibit a more cardiac-restricted phenotype with fibrofatty degeneration of the myocardium and it is conducting system. More than 200 different lamin A/C (LMNA) mutations are associated with inherited cardiomyopathy, primarily DCM that may be associated with conduction system disease prior to the evidence of ventricular dilatation due to fibrofatty degeneration of the myocardium and conducting cells [52, 55]. Other diseases caused by lamin A/C mutations are Charcot-Marie-Tooth neuropathy, Dunningan partial familial lipodystrophy, progeria and other overlapping syndromes, all known as laminopathies [63].

#### *2.4.2.6 Ion channel*

The function of sarcolemmal transmembrane cardiac voltage-gated sodium channel is crucial in the generation of cardiac action potentials. Some mutations in the encoding gene SCNA5 are implicated in DCM. SCN5A mutations causes high burden of arrhythmias. There are also many allelic variants in SCN5A, including those leading to Brugada syndrome, idiopathic ventricular fibrillation (VF), familial atrial fibrillation (AF), left ventricular non-compaction cardiomyopathy, and long QT syndrome type III [54, 59, 64].

#### *2.4.2.7 Extracellular matrix-cell-adhesion and signaling*

Extracellular matrix proteins such as laminin alpha-4 (LAMA4) and Fukutin (FKTN) have been described in relation to DCM. They may lead to DCM phenotype by disrupting signaling pathways and modifying cell-surface molecules [50].

The genetic evaluation of DCM is summarized in **Table 2**.

| Genetic evaluation of DCM | Gene screening of DCM | Genotype correlations of DCM |
|---|---|---|
| Sarcomere protein related genes | • Titin (TNN)<br>• α-Cardiac actin (ACTC 1 and ACTC 2)<br>• α-Tropomyosin 1 (TPM 1)<br>• Cardiac troponin subtypes (TNNT2, TNNC1, TNNI3)<br>• Myosin heavy chains (MYH 6, MYH7)<br>• Myosin-binding protein C (MYBPC)<br>• Troponin I-interacting kinase (TNNI3K) | • 12–25% of genetic related DCM are associated with titin (TTN) mutations<br>• α-Tropomyosin 1 (TPM 1) mutations are described in 1–2% of DCM<br>• Myosin heavy chain (MYH7)-mutations in 3–4% of DCM<br>• 3% of DCM are linked to cardiac troponin T (TNNT2) mutations<br>• Gene defects in sarcomere proteins are associated with defects in force generation and transmission<br>• TNNI3K-mutations may cause conduction defects and atrial fibrillation |
| Cytoskeletal protein related genes: Z-disc Dystrophin complex Cytoskeleton | • α-Actinin 2 (ACTN 2)<br>• Muscle LIM protein (MLP)<br>• Cysteine- and glycine-rich protein 3 (CSPR3)<br>• Telethonin (TCAP)<br>• Cypher/Z-band (LDB3)<br>• PDZ LIM domain protein 3 (PDLIM3)<br>• Cardiac ankyrin repeat protein (CARP)<br>• Myopalladin (MYPN)<br>• Nexilin (NEXN)<br>• Metavinculin (VCL)<br>• Dystrophin (DMD)<br>• Sacroglycan (SGCA, SGCB, SGCD, and SGCG)<br>• Desmin (DES) | • Metavinculin (CVL) mutations are related to 1% of DCM<br>• Dystrophin (DMD) mutations are associated with Duchenne/Becker muscular dystrophy<br>• Sacroglycan (SDC) mutations can cause Limb-girdle-muscular dystrophy<br>Prevalence of *Desmin (DES)* mutations in genetic related DCM is about 1–2%, the mutations are often related with myofibrillar myopathy, ARCV and cardiac conduction blocks |
| Desmosomal protein related genes | • Plakoglobin (JUP)<br>• Desmoplakin (DSP)<br>• Desmocollin 2 (DSC2)<br>• Desmoglein 2 (DSG2)<br>• Plakophilin-2 (PKP2) | • Mutations in desmosomal genes are frequent in patients with advanced DCM undergoing cardiac transplantation<br>• Desmosomal gene mutations are also linked to ARVC<br>• Desmoplakin (DSP) causes 2% of genetic related DCM<br>• Plakoglobin (JUP)-mutations are also associated with Naxos syndrome<br>• Desmocollin 2 (DSC2) mutations may lead to mild palmoplantar keratoderma |
| Sarcoplasmic reticulum related genes | • Ryanodine receptor 2 (RyR2)<br>• Phospholamban (PLN)<br>• SR proteins, Ca-ATPase pump (SERCA2a) | • Specific mutations are associated with high risk of malignant ventricular arrhythmias and end-stage heart failure<br>• Ryanodine receptor 2 (RyR2) correlates with cathecolaminergic polymorphic ventricular tachycardia and ARVC<br>• Phospholamban (PLN) mutations can cause ARVC<br>• Some other genes encoding for sarcoplasmic reticulum and cytoplasm related proteins like PTPN11, RAF1 and RIT1 are also associated with Noonan and Leopard Syndrome |

| Genetic evaluation of DCM | Gene screening of DCM | Genotype correlations of DCM |
|---|---|---|
| Nuclear envelope and nucleus protein related genes | • Emerin (EMD)<br>• Lamin A/C (LMNA) | • EMD mutations can lead to X-linked Emery-Dreyfuss muscular dystrophy, joint contractures and conduction system disease<br>• Prevalence of genetic-related DCM due to LMNA mutation is described in 4–8%<br>• LMNA-related heart failure is often more resistant to heart failure therapy and has a high risk for arrhythmias and sudden cardiac death<br>• Mutations in LMNA can cause a severe and progressive DCM and can also lead to Charcot-Marie-Tooth neuropathy, Dunningan partial familial lipodystrophy, Emery-Dreyfuss muscular dystrophy and progeria |
| Ion channel protein related genes | • Sodium channel, voltage-gated, type V, alpha subunit (SCNA5)<br>• Potassium channel (KCNQ1) | • *SCN5A* mutations account for 2–3% of DCM, mutations are associated with Brugada syndrome, Long QT syndrome, atrial fibrillation and conduction defects<br>• KCNQ1 mutations may induce atrial fibrillation, Long QT 1, Short QT1 and Jervell and Lange-Nielsen syndrome |
| Extracellular matrix protein related genes | • Laminin alpha-4 (LAMA4)<br>• Fukutin (FKTN) | • Extracellular matrix protein relation has been described to DCM<br>• FKTN and LAMA2 mutations can also cause congenital muscular dystrophy |

**Table 2.**
*Genetic aspects of dilated cardiomyopathy.*

## 2.5 Diagnosis

Establishing the etiology is of great importance as it may influence treatment and prognosis of patients with DCM. Beside the conventional clinical tools, modern imaging and genetic tools are available to elucidate and ensure the correct diagnosis. The recently published statement for the diagnostic workup on DCM from the ESC working group on myocardial and pericardial diseases recommend the following steps: first the diagnostic evaluation should be start with in-depth personal and family history, followed by physical examination, an electrocardiogram (ECG), and echocardiography [8]. These steps often sufficiently differentiate between acquired and familial DCM. If there is no suspicion of an acquired DCM and if ‘red flags’ are recognized, the second-level diagnostic work-up should be added. ‘Red flags’ are defined as signs and suspicion on a specific etiology. Biochemical analyses, cardiac magnetic resonance imaging (CMR), endomyocardial biopsy (EMB), and genetic testing are recommended in a second step. However, the patient’s age plays a crucial role in the decision-making during the diagnostic procedure and should be rated against the potential benefit of dedicated investigations. The detailed diagnostic workup and possible red flags are presented in **Table 3**.

## 2.6 Screening

In common, DCM is a slowly progressive disease and screening is essential for an early diagnosis of asymptomatic family members. Currently, screening all first-degree family members of patients with genetic proven or non-genetic forms of DCM with a positive family history is recommended. The screening comprises

| Diagnostic tool | Look for | Red flags for specific disorders |
|---|---|---|
| Personal and familial history | Degree of symptoms<br>Travel history<br>Inheritance pattern<br>Toxin exposition Involvement of other organs | Intellectual and sensorineural disabilities<br>Muscle weakness<br>Myotonia<br>Gait disturbances<br>Skin abnormities, for example, hyperpigmentation and palmoplantar keratoderma, butterfly-shaped face rash<br>Woolly hair |
| Electrocardiogram | | Low P-wave amplitude<br>Atrioventricular block<br>Repolarization disorders with non-coronary distribution<br>Low QRS amplitude<br>Bundle branch block<br>Long QTc<br>Ventricular arrhythmias |
| 24 h electrocardiogram | Relevant brady- and tachyarrhythmias | Relevant tachyarrhythmias |
| 24 h ambulatory blood pressure monitoring | Exclude persistent hypertension | |
| Biochemistry | Blood count<br>Electrolytes<br>Renal function<br>Cardiac biomarkers<br>TSH<br>HbA1c<br>Serum iron, ferritin and electrophoresis<br>Urine chemistry and proteinuria<br>Serum free light chains<br>HIV and hepatitis serology<br>Other specific serology tests in accordance symptoms and clinical suspicion | High levels of creatine kinase<br>Myoglobinuria<br>Increased serum iron & ferritin levels<br>Leucopenia or neutropenia<br>Free light chains for amyloidosis<br>Diabetes and lactatacidosis<br>Thyroid disorders<br>Infectious etiologies |
| Echocardiography | Ventricular dilatation<br>Valve diseases<br>Right ventricular pathologies | Left ventricular hypertrabecularisation<br>Segmental dysfunction with noncoronary distribution |
| Coronary angiography | Exclude coronary artery disease | |
| CMR | Late Gadolinium Enhancement<br>Intramyocardial edema<br>Intramyocardial iron deposit<br>Right ventricular morphology<br>Molly sequence | Patchy or inferobasal late gadolinium enhancement (LGE) distribution<br>"Midwall sign" septal wall LGE distribution |
| EBM | Giant cell myocarditis | |
| Genetics | Screening familial DCM | |

**Table 3.**
*Diagnostic workup and possible red flags in dilated cardiomyopathy.*

physical examination, 12-lead ECG and transthoracic echocardiography as well as measurement of CK levels. The CK levels may help to identify subclinical skeletal muscle abnormalities and to provide supportive evidence for the presence of an inherited myopathy. If DCM is suspected in first-degree relatives, the screening should be repeated anually. Otherwise, asymptomatic first-degree relatives should be rescreened at three- to five-year intervals because of possible late onset of DCM phenotype [21].

## 2.7 Therapy

Specific treatment is applicable in syndrome associated DCM, for example, infectious etiologies and infiltrative disorders. However, specific treatment is not available for most DCM patients. Therefore, the therapy focuses on improvement of clinical symptoms as well as on the control of disease progression and potential complications such as sudden cardiac arrest.

### *2.7.1 Heart failure treatment*

Guidelines recommend the following treatment for acute HF, not including non-cardiogenic shock: oxygen, non-invasive ventilation (NIV), intravenous diuretics (20–40 mg bolus furosemide at admission), and intravenous nitrates. Intravenous nitrates have long been described to improve hemodynamic and dyspnea in HF patients by many ways: decrease in systemic blood pressure and left ventricular afterload, substantial reduction preload and therefore of in right and left ventricular filling pressure, an increase in cardiac output, and little or no change in heart rate [65]. Improvement in cardiac output by intravenous nitrates is mostly related to the reduction in left ventricular afterload, but is also influenced by a decrease in pulmonary vascular resistance, improvement in myocardial oxygenation, and a reduction of mitral regurgitation. Administration of inotropes and/or vasopressors is recommended in patients with signs of low cardiac output [66]. However, application of inotropes and/or vasopressors is associated with an increased long-term mortality risk [67–69]. Additional treatment includes the optimal dosing of angiotensin-converting enzyme inhibitors (ACEI) or angiotensin receptor blockers (ARB). ACEI have been shown to reduce cardiovascular mortality and prevent rehospitalization in patients with HF in two key randomized controlled trails (CONSENSUS and SOLVD-Treatment) [70]. Likewise, ARB improve long-term outcome in HF patients [71]. Another essential component of HF therapy is spironolactone. The RALES study has shown a reduction in mortality after addition of 25 mg of spironolactone to the standard treatment in HF patients with an LVEF <35% [72]. The international guidelines recommend spironolactone in all patients presenting with moderate to severe HF symptoms. In the PARADIGM-HF trial, the use of angiotensin receptor-neprilysin inhibitor (ARNI) (sacubitril/valsartan) showed a reduction of the composite endpoint of cardiovascular death or HF hospitalization by 20% compared with enalapril alone in symptomatic HF patients with reduced LVEF [73]. These study results are implemented in the updated ACC/AHA/HFSA guidelines on management of HF, which recommend to replace ACEI or ARB by sacubitril/valsartan in patients with reduced LVEF and ongoing symptoms [74]. Betablockers reduce mortality in HF patients even without reduced ejection fraction as has been demonstrated by multicenter placebo-controlled studies [75–77]. Because of the negative inotropic effect of betablockers, patients should not be treated in the very acute presentation with signs or symptoms of decompensation and initial doses should be low. Long-term goal is a heart rate below 70 bpm in sinus rhythm. If this is not obtainable with the maximum, or maximum tolerated dose of betablockers, the current European heart failure guidelines recommend the addition of Ivabradine [66]. In addition to pharmacological medication cardiac resynchronization therapy (CRT) has been shown to improve cardiac performance, to reduce symptoms, morbidity, and mortality [78, 79].

### *2.7.2 Anticoagulation*

The role of anticoagulation in DCM with sinus rhythm is unclear [80]. The prospective randomized trials were either underpowered or with a too short follow-up. At present, there are no trial data to guide anticoagulant treatment regime in DCM. Due to two studies (WATCH and WARCEF trial) showing a slight advantage of warfarin over aspirin, anticoagulation with warfarin is advised in patients with a history of thromboembolism or evidence of intracardiac thrombus [81, 82]. Current ACC/AHA HF guidelines do not recommend anticoagulation in reduced left ventricular function and sinus rhythm without prior thromboembolic events or known cardioembolic source [83]. Studies testing the non-vitamin K antagonist oral anticoagulants (NOACs) in patients with reduced left ventricular function are currently ongoing. In DCM patients with documented AF, oral anticoagulant is recommended with $CHA_2DS_2$-VASc score $\geq 2$, as a class I indication and in men with a $CHA_2DS_2$-VASc score of 1 as class IIa with level of evidence B [66, 77, 83, 84].

*2.7.3 Arrhythmias*

The most common arrhythmia in DCM is AF, which increases the risk of thromboembolic complications, impairs cardiac function and worsening HF symptoms. Therefore, evaluation of rate control and anticoagulation in order to preserve LV-function and prevent thromboembolic events is crucial. In the acute setting betablockers, digoxin and their combination may be used to control ventricular rate. In the chronic stage, rhythm control has been shown to be superior to rate control alone in reducing mortality [85]. Because of the commonly reduced left ventricular function, the only therapeutic option is type III antiarrhythmic drug such as amiodarone. Alternatively, electrical cardioversion can be performed. Recently, the CASTLE-AF study demonstrated the superiority of AF catheter ablation in certain patients with HF as compared to medical therapy. The ablation was associated with a significantly lower rate of death and hospitalization for worsening HF [86]. DCM patients may suffer from ventricular arrhythmias (VA), which are mainly caused by myocardial damage, fibrosis and/or loss of cell-to-cell conjunctions, that are described by three mechanisms: reentry, trigger activity, and automatism [87]. Monomorphic ventricular tachycardias (VTs) are frequently induced by macro-reentry mechanism, which is best treated by ablation. The main trigger mechanisms are electrolyte imbalance, mostly secondary to diuretic treatment, antiarrhythmic drugs, and bradycardia. The therapeutic options are a combination of antiarrhythmic drugs like betablockers and type III antiarrhythmics and/or implantation of an implantable cardioverter defibrillator (ICD). The indications for ICD treatment are described later [4].

### 2.8 Prognosis and risk stratification

Although there has been a significant improvement in prognosis of DCM patients over the last decades, mortality is still high. The prognosis is mainly influenced by HF symptoms and more relevant by the appearance of VTs. Survival data of adults with DCM have shown a one-year mortality of 25–30% and a 50% survival at 5 years. Sustained VT or VF presents the main cause for SCD, which occurs in up to 12% of DCM patients [4, 88]. In general, the prevalence of sustained VT (monomorphic or polymorphic) is estimated as less than 5% [89]. Recently, the Pediatric Cardiomyopathy Registry presented a 5-year incidence rate of SCD in children with DCM of 3% [90]. An age at diagnosis below 14 years, LV dilation, and posterior wall thinning were identified as the most important risk factors. In contrast, the mortality in adults is mostly associated with age and male gender, reduced New York Heart Association (NYHA) functional class, impaired LVEF, and the presence of specific cardiac biomarkers as well as myocardial fibrosis in CMR [91–94]. Furthermore, genetic aspects play an important role for detection of high-risk patients. Most commonly the pathogenic mutation in the lamin A/C (LMNA) gene is associated with atrial and ventricular arrhythmias. LMNA mutation has been identified as the most malignant and penetrant condition with worse outcomes compared to other forms of DCM [95]. Beside risk models such as the Seattle Heart Failure Model for the prediction of prognosis in the general population of HF patients, there exist no specific risk tools for DCM patients [96]. For the identification of high-risk DCM patients, a personalized and precise approach is required (**Table 3**). This should include the personal and familial history, measurement of LVEF, detailed search for VA and proof of fibrosis using CMR. Other promising approaches are expected to be helpful in decision-making in high-risk DCM patients, determination of microvolt T-wave alternans analysis and detection of autonomic dysfunction using nuclear imaging. In addition, detection of LMNA gene mutation has been described to identify the high-risk DCM population. However, all these approaches need further research.

### 2.9 Prevention of sudden cardiac death

The most effective therapy of malignant VTs and thus prevention of SCD in DCM patients is the implantation of an ICD. Current ESC guidelines recommend the implantation of a defibrillator in patients who experienced VT or VF (secondary prevention of sudden cardiac death), as well as in high risk patients for primary prevention. The latter are patients with symptomatic HF NYHA class II–III and LVEF ≤35% after ≥3 months of optimal medical therapy who are expected to survive for at least 1 year [97]. Similarly, the American College of Cardiology and American Heart Association guidelines recommend ICD therapy in patients with LVEF ≤35% due to prior myocardial infarction (MI), at least 40 days post-MI, or non-ischemic DCM and NYHA class II or III [98]. However, existing guidelines lack sensitivity and specificity for the selection of patients with DCM for primary prevention ICD implantation. A recently presented meta-analysis by Golwala et al. has demonstrated a 23% reduction in all-cause mortality with ICD therapy compared with optimal medical therapy alone (HR, 0.77; 95% CI, 0.64–0.91) [99]. Although ICD implantation seems to be the best possible option for SCD prevention in DCM, there remain potential complications. Inappropriate shocks, risk of infection, device or lead replacement have to be considered and discussed in detail before an ICD is implanted.

## 3. Conclusion

DCM includes a heterogeneous group of myocardial and systemic conditions causing left ventricular dilatation and dysfunction. DCM is one of the most common cardiomyopathies worldwide. Yet, the real prevalence is unknown. The etiology contains non-genetic (e.g. myocarditis, peripartum, toxics, arrhythmia, infiltrative etiologies, endocrine, nutritional, and neuromuscular) and genetic causes. Literature on genetic mutations being responsible for DCM has increased exponentially. Today, up to 30% of the DCM cases are described to be caused by a gene mutation, the majority of which occur in autosomal genes that encode for a wide range of proteins of the cardiomyocyte's structural elements. Mutations in genes encoding sarcomeric, cytoskeletal, desmosomal, nuclear membrane, mitochondrial, and RNA-binding proteins have all been linked to DCM. However, the most common mutations occur in genes encoding sarcomeric proteins and in genes related to the nuclear envelope and the cytoskeleton. Therefore, the diagnostic workup of DCM should involve the clinical tools as well as imaging and gen-technologies. Specific treatment is only available for syndrome-associated DCM. The majority of the DCM patients are treated for HF symptoms, prevention of thromboembolic events, and malign arrhythmias. The prognosis of DCM patients is variable and depends on multiple risk factors. Some, for example, LVEF and NYHA functional class are known for years as risk factors of SCD, others need further research before they can be established in clinical routine.

## Conflict of interest

The authors declare no conflict of interest.

## Acronyms and abbreviations

| | |
|---|---|
| ACEI | angiotensin converting enzyme inhibitors |
| AF | atrial fibrillation |
| AIDS | acquired immune deficiency syndrome |
| AHA | American Heart Association |
| ARB | angiotensin receptor blockers |
| ARVC | arrhythmogenic right ventricular cardiomyopathy |
| CAD | coronary artery disease |
| CARP | cardiac ankyrin repeat protein |
| CK | creatine kinase |
| CMR | cardiac magnetic resonance imaging |
| DCM | dilated cardiomyopathy |
| DES | desmin |
| ECG | electrocardiogram |
| EMB | endomyocardial biopsy |
| ESC | European Society of Cardiology |
| HCM | hypertrophic cardiomyopathy |
| HF | heart failure |
| HIV | human immundeficiency virus |
| ICD | implantable cardioverter defibrillator |
| IDC | idiopathic dilated cardiomyopathy |
| ISFC | International Society and Federation of Cardiology |
| LAMA4 | laminin alpha-4 |
| LINC | links the nucleus to the cytoplasm |
| LMNA | lamin A/C |
| LVEF | left ventricular ejection fraction |
| MI | myocardial infarction |
| MLP | muscle LIM protein |
| MYH | myosin proteins |
| NCCM | non-compaction cardiomyopathy |
| NIV | non-invasive ventilation |
| NOAC | non-vitamin K antagonist oral anticoagulant |
| NYHA | New York Heart Association |
| PPCM | peripartum cardiomyopathy |
| RCM | restrictive cardiomyopathy |
| RNA | ribonucleid acid |
| RyR2 | ryanodine receptor 2 |

| | |
|---|---|
| SCD | sudden cardiac death |
| TPM | troponin-tropomyosin |
| TNN | cardiac troponin |
| VA/VT/VF | ventricular arrhythmia/ventricular tachycardia/ventricular fibrillation |
| WHO | World Health Organization |

## Author details

Deborah P. Schild, Sascha I. Ricciardi, Jens G. Hellige, Rolf Vogel and Nisha Arenja*
Department of Cardiology, Solothurner Spitäler AG, Kantonsspital Olten and Bürgerspital Solothurn, Switzerland

*Address all correspondence to: nisha.arenja@spital.so.ch

## References


[1] Towbin JA et al. Incidence, causes, and outcomes of dilated cardiomyopathy in children. JAMA. 2006;**296**(15):1867-1876

[2] Richardson P et al. Report of the 1995 World Health Organization/ International Society and Federation of Cardiology Task Force on the definition and classification of cardiomyopathies. Circulation. 1996;**93**(5):841-842

[3] Elliott P, Andersson B, Arbustini E, Bilinska Z, Cecchi F, Charron P, et al. Classification of the cardiomyopathies: A position statement from the European society of cardiology workring group on myocardial and pericardial diseases. European Heart Journal. 2008;**29**:270-276

[4] Dec GW, Fuster V. Idiopathic dilated cardiomyopathy. The New England Journal of Medicine. 1994;**331**(23):1564-1575

[5] Givertz MM, Mann DL. Epidemiology and natural history of recovery of left ventricular function in recent onset dilated cardiomyopathies. Current Heart Failure Reports. 2013;**10**(4):321-330

[6] Report of the WHO/ISFC task force on the definition and classification of cardiomyopathies. British Heart Journal. 1980;**44**(6):672-673

[7] Maron BJ et al. Contemporary definitions and classification of the cardiomyopathies: An American Heart Association Scientific Statement from the Council on Clinical Cardiology, Heart Failure and Transplantation Committee; Quality of Care and Outcomes Research and Functional Genomics and Translational Biology Interdisciplinary Working Groups; and Council on Epidemiology and Prevention. Circulation. 2006;**113**(14):1807-1816

[8] Pinto YM et al. Proposal for a revised definition of dilated cardiomyopathy, hypokinetic non-dilated cardiomyopathy, and its implications for clinical practice: A position statement of the ESC working group on myocardial and pericardial diseases. European Heart Journal. 2016;**37**(23):1850-1858

[9] Codd MB et al. Epidemiology of idiopathic dilated and hypertrophic cardiomyopathy. A population-based study in Olmsted County, Minnesota, 1975-1984. Circulation. 1989;**80**(3):564-572

[10] Hershberger RE, Hedges DJ, Morales A. Dilated cardiomyopathy: The complexity of a diverse genetic architecture. Nature Reviews. Cardiology. 2013;**10**(9):531-547

[11] Burkett EL, Hershberger RE. Clinical and genetic issues in familial dilated cardiomyopathy. Journal of the American College of Cardiology. 2005;**45**(7):969-981

[12] Ganesh SK et al. Genetics and genomics for the prevention and treatment of cardiovascular disease: Update: A scientific statement from the American Heart Association. Circulation. 2013;**128**(25):2813-2851

[13] Mestroni L et al. Guidelines for the study of familial dilated cardiomyopathies. Collaborative Research Group of the European Human and Capital Mobility Project on Familial Dilated Cardiomyopathy. European Heart Journal. 1999;**20**(2):93-102

[14] Gavazzi A et al. Evidence-based diagnosis of familial non-X-linked dilated cardiomyopathy. Prevalence, inheritance and characteristics. European Heart Journal. 2001;**22**(1):73-81

[15] Goerss JB et al. Frequency of familial dilated cardiomyopathy.

European Heart Journal. 1995;**16**(Suppl O):2-4

[16] Grunig E et al. Frequency and phenotypes of familial dilated cardiomyopathy. Journal of the American College of Cardiology. 1998;**31**(1):186-194

[17] Mahon NG et al. Echocardiographic evaluation in asymptomatic relatives of patients with dilated cardiomyopathy reveals preclinical disease. Annals of Internal Medicine. 2005;**143**(2):108-115

[18] Mestroni L et al. Familial dilated cardiomyopathy: Evidence for genetic and phenotypic heterogeneity. Journal of the American College of Cardiology. 1999;**34**(1):181-190. Heart Muscle Disease Study Group

[19] Pogwizd SM, McKenzie JP, Cain ME. Mechanisms underlying spontaneous and induced ventricular arrhythmias in patients with idiopathic dilated cardiomyopathy. Circulation. 1998;**98**(22):2404-2414

[20] Bakalakos A, Ritsatos K, Anastasakis A. Current perspectives on the diagnosis and management of dilated cardiomyopathy beyond heart failure: A cardiomyopathy clinic doctor's point of view. Hellenic Journal of Cardiology. 2018. https://doi.org/10.1016/j.hjc.2018.05.008

[21] Hershberger RE et al. Genetic evaluation of cardiomyopathy—A Heart Failure Society of America practice guideline. Journal of Cardiac Failure. 2009;**15**(2):83-97

[22] Taylor MR, Carniel E, Mestroni L. Cardiomyopathy, familial dilated. Orphanet Journal of Rare Diseases. 2006;**1**:27

[23] Hazebroek M, Dennert R, Heymans S. Idiopathic dilated cardiomyopathy: Possible triggers and treatment strategies. Netherlands Heart Journal. 2012;**20**(7-8):332-335

[24] Weintraub RG, Semsarian C, Macdonald P. Dilated cardiomyopathy. Lancet. 2017;**390**(10092):400-414

[25] Dennert R, Crijns HJ, Heymans S. Acute viral myocarditis. European Heart Journal. 2008;**29**(17):2073-2082

[26] Bozkurt B et al. Current diagnostic and treatment strategies for specific dilated cardiomyopathies: A scientific statement from the American Heart Association. Circulation. 2016;**134**(23):e579-e646

[27] Wendt S et al. Brucella related myocarditis. International Journal of Infectious Diseases. 2018;**66**:126-127

[28] Villablanca P et al. Salmonella berta myocarditis: Case report and systematic review of non-typhoid Salmonella myocarditis. World Journal of Cardiology. 2015;**7**(12):931-937

[29] Samdani S et al. Cardiac complications in diphtheria and predictors of outcomes. International Journal of Pediatric Otorhinolaryngology. 2018;**104**:76-78

[30] Diaz F, Collazos J. Myopericarditis due to Chlamydia psittaci. The role of autoimmunity. Scandinavian Journal of Infectious Diseases. 1997;**29**(1):93-94

[31] Komuro J et al. Various cardiac abnormalities caused by bacterial myocarditis. International Heart Journal. 2018;**59**(1):229-232

[32] Cunha BA et al. Lyme carditis with isolated left bundle branch block and myocarditis successfully treated with oral doxycycline. IDCases. 2018;**11**:48-50

[33] Rassi A Jr, Rassi A, Little WC. Chagas' heart disease. Clinical Cardiology. 2000;**23**(12):883-889

[34] Elkayam U et al. Pregnancy-associated cardiomyopathy: Clinical

characteristics and a comparison between early and late presentation. Circulation. 2005;**111**(16):2050-2055

[35] Regitz-Zagrosek V et al. ESC guidelines for the management of cardiovascular diseases during pregnancy. European Heart Journal. 2018;**2018, 39**(34):3165-3241

[36] Ntusi NB, Mayosi BM. Aetiology and risk factors of peripartum cardiomyopathy: A systematic review. International Journal of Cardiology. 2009;**131**(2):168-179

[37] van Spaendonck-Zwarts KY, van Tintelen JP, van Veldhuisen DJ, van der Werf R, Jongbloed JD, Paulus WJ, et al. Peripartum cardiomyopathy as a part of familial dilated cardiomyopathy. Circulation. 2010;**121**:2169-2175

[38] Sisakian H. Cardiomyopathies: Evolution of pathogenesis concepts and potential for new therapies. World Journal of Cardiology. 2014;**6**(6):478-494

[39] Piano MR. Alcoholic cardiomyopathy: Incidence, clinical characteristics, and pathophysiology. Chest. 2002;**121**(5):1638-1650

[40] Higgins AY, O'Halloran TD, Chang JD. Chemotherapy-induced cardiomyopathy. Heart Failure Reviews. 2015;**20**(6):721-730

[41] Figueredo VM. Chemical cardiomyopathies: The negative effects of medications and nonprescribed drugs on the heart. The American Journal of Medicine. 2011;**124**(6):480-488

[42] Gossage AM, Braxton Hicks JA. On auricular fibrillation. The Quarterly Journal of Medicine. 1913;**6**:435-440

[43] Le Lan C et al. Redox active plasma iron in C282Y/C282Y hemochromatosis. Blood. 2005;**105**(11):4527-4531

[44] Bhogal S et al. Cardiac amyloidosis: An updated review with emphasis on diagnosis and future directions. Current Problems in Cardiology. 2018;**43**(1):10-34

[45] Klein I, Danzi S. Thyroid disease and the heart. Circulation. 2007;**116**(15):1725-1735

[46] Rubis P. The diagnostic work up of genetic and inflammatory dilated cardiomyopathy. e-Journal of the ESC Council for Cardiology Practice. 2015;**13**(19)

[47] Munguti CM, Al Rifai M, Shaheen W. A rare cause of cardiomyopathy: A case of selenium deficiency causing severe cardiomyopathy that improved on supplementation. Cureus. 2017;**9**(8):e1627

[48] Kothari SS, Sharma M. L-carnitine in children with idiopathic dilated cardiomyopathy. Indian Heart Journal. 1998;**50**(1):59-61

[49] Watkins H, Ashrafian H, Redwood C. Inherited cardiomyopathies. The New England Journal of Medicine. 2011;**364**(17):1643-1656

[50] Mestroni L et al. Genetic causes of dilated cardiomyopathy. Progress in Pediatric Cardiology. 2014;**37**(1-2):13-18

[51] McNally EM, Mestroni L. Dilated cardiomyopathy: Genetic determinants and mechanisms. Circulation Research. 2017;**121**(7):731-748

[52] McNally EM, Golbus JR, Puckelwartz MJ. Genetic mutations and mechanisms in dilated cardiomyopathy. The Journal of Clinical Investigation. 2013;**123**(1):19-26

[53] Garfinkel AC, Seidman JG, Seidman CE. Genetic pathogenesis of hypertrophic and dilated cardiomyopathy. Heart Failure Clinics. 2018;**14**(2):139-146

[54] Burke MA et al. Clinical and mechanistic insights into the genetics of cardiomyopathy. Journal of the American College of Cardiology. 2016;**68**(25):2871-2886

[55] Morita H, Seidman J, Seidman CE. Genetic causes of human heart failure. The Journal of Clinical Investigation. 2005;**115**(3):518-526

[56] Lee HJ, Zheng JJ. PDZ domains and their binding partners: Structure, specificity, and modification. Cell Communication and Signaling: CCS. 2010;**8**:8

[57] Towbin JA et al. X-linked dilated cardiomyopathy. Molecular genetic evidence of linkage to the Duchenne muscular dystrophy (dystrophin) gene at the Xp21 locus. Circulation. 1993;**87**(6):1854-1865

[58] Tsikitis M et al. Intermediate filaments in cardiomyopathy. Biophysical Reviews. 2018;**10**(4):1007-1031

[59] Dellefave L, McNally EM. The genetics of dilated cardiomyopathy. Current Opinion in Cardiology. 2010;**25**(3):198-204

[60] Taylor MR et al. Prevalence of desmin mutations in dilated cardiomyopathy. Circulation. 2007;**115**(10):1244-1251

[61] Cho Y. Arrhythmogenic right ventricular cardiomyopathy. Journal of Arrhythmia. 2018;**34**:356-368

[62] van Rijsingen IA et al. Outcome in phospholamban R14del carriers: Results of a large multicentre cohort study. Circulation. Cardiovascular Genetics. 2014;**7**(4):455-465

[63] Goidescu CM. Dilated cardiomyopathy produced by lamin A/C gene mutations. Clujul Medical. 2013;**86**(4):309-312

[64] Liu Y, Chen H, Shou W. Potential common pathogenic pathways for the left ventricular noncompaction cardiomyopathy (LVNC). Pediatric Cardiology. 2018;**39**(6):1099-1106

[65] Gogia H et al. Prevention of tolerance to hemodynamic effects of nitrates with concomitant use of hydralazine in patients with chronic heart failure. Journal of the American College of Cardiology. 1995;**26**(7):1575-1580

[66] Ponikowski P et al. ESC Guidelines for the diagnosis and treatment of acute and chronic heart failure: The task force for the diagnosis and treatment of acute and chronic heart failure of the European Society of Cardiology (ESC) developed with the special contribution of the Heart Failure Association (HFA) of the ESC. European Heart Journal. 2016;**2016, 37**(27):2129-2200

[67] Mebazaa A et al. Long-term safety of intravenous cardiovascular agents in acute heart failure: Results from the European Society of Cardiology Heart Failure Long-Term Registry. European Journal of Heart Failure. 2018;**20**(2):332-341

[68] Mebazaa A et al. Short-term survival by treatment among patients hospitalized with acute heart failure: The global ALARM-HF registry using propensity scoring methods. Intensive Care Medicine. 2011;**37**(2):290-301

[69] Mortara A et al. Treatment with inotropes and related prognosis in acute heart failure: Contemporary data from the Italian Network on Heart Failure (IN-HF) Outcome registry. The Journal of Heart and Lung Transplantation. 2014;**33**(10):1056-1065

[70] Group, C.T.S. Effects of enalapril on mortality in severe congestive heart failure. Results of the Cooperative North Scandinavian Enalapril Survival Study (CONSENSUS). The New England

Journal of Medicine. 1987;**316**(23):1429-1435

[71] Cohn JN et al. Rationale and design of the valsartan heart failure trial: A large multinational trial to assess the effects of valsartan, an angiotensin-receptor blocker, on morbidity and mortality in chronic congestive heart failure. Journal of Cardiac Failure. 1999;**5**(2):155-160

[72] Pitt B et al. The effect of spironolactone on morbidity and mortality in patients with severe heart failure. Randomized Aldactone Evaluation Study Investigators. The New England Journal of Medicine. 1999;**341**(10):709-717

[73] McMurray JJ et al. Angiotensin-neprilysin inhibition versus enalapril in heart failure. The New England Journal of Medicine. 2014;**371**(11):993-1004

[74] Yancy CW et al. 2016 ACC/AHA/HFSA Focused Update on New Pharmacological Therapy for Heart Failure: An Update of the 2013 ACCF/AHA Guideline for the Management of Heart Failure: A Report of the American College of Cardiology/American Heart Association Task Force on Clinical Practice Guidelines and the Heart Failure Society of America. Journal of the American College of Cardiology. 2016;**68**(13):1476-1488

[75] Packer M et al. The effect of carvedilol on morbidity and mortality in patients with chronic heart failure. U.S. Carvedilol Heart Failure Study Group. The New England Journal of Medicine. 1996;**334**(21):1349-1355

[76] CIBIS-II Investigators and Committees. The cardiac insufficiency bisoprolol study II (CIBIS-II): A randomised trial. Lancet. 1999;**353**(9146):9-13

[77] MERITHF Study Group. Effect of metoprolol CR/XL in chronic heart failure: Metoprolol CR/XL randomised Intervention Trial in Congestive Heart Failure (MERIT-HF). Lancet. 1999;**353**(9169):2001-2007

[78] Sohaib SM et al. Opportunity to increase life span in narrow QRS cardiac resynchronization therapy recipients by deactivating ventricular pacing: Evidence from randomized controlled trials. JACC: Heart Failure. 2015;**3**(4):327-336

[79] Tang AS et al. Cardiac-resynchronization therapy for mild-to-moderate heart failure. The New England Journal of Medicine. 2010;**363**(25):2385-2395

[80] Mischie AN et al. Anticoagulation in patients with dilated cardiomyopathy, low ejection fraction, and sinus rhythm: Back to the drawing board. Cardiovascular Therapeutics. 2013;**31**(5):298-302

[81] Massie BM et al. Randomized trial of warfarin, aspirin, and clopidogrel in patients with chronic heart failure: The Warfarin and Antiplatelet Therapy in Chronic Heart Failure (WATCH) trial. Circulation. 2009;**119**(12):1616-1624

[82] Homma S et al. Warfarin and aspirin in patients with heart failure and sinus rhythm. The New England Journal of Medicine. 2012;**366**(20):1859-1869

[83] Yancy CW et al. 2013 ACCF/AHA guideline for the management of heart failure: A report of the American College of Cardiology Foundation/American Heart Association Task Force on Practice Guidelines. Journal of the American College of Cardiology. 2013;**62**(16):e147-e239

[84] Kirchhof P et al. ESC Guidelines for the management of atrial fibrillation developed in collaboration with EACTS. European Heart Journal. 2016;**37**(38):2893-2962

[85] Roy D et al. Rhythm control versus rate control for atrial fibrillation and

heart failure. The New England Journal of Medicine. 2008;**358**(25):2667-2677

[86] Marrouche NF et al. Catheter ablation for atrial fibrillation with heart failure. The New England Journal of Medicine. 2018;**378**(5):417-427

[87] Merino JL. Mechanisms underlying ventricular arrhythmias in idiopathic dilated cardiomyopathy: Implications for management. American Journal of Cardiovascular Drugs. 2001;**1**(2):105-118

[88] Milner PG, Dimarco JP, Lerman BB. Electrophysiological evaluation of sustained ventricular tachyarrhythmias in idiopathic dilated cardiomyopathy. Pacing and Clinical Electrophysiology. 1988;**11**(5):562-568

[89] Teerlink JR et al. Ambulatory ventricular arrhythmias in patients with heart failure do not specifically predict an increased risk of sudden death. PROMISE (Prospective Randomized Milrinone Survival Evaluation) Investigators. Circulation. 2000;**101**(1):40-46

[90] Pahl E et al. Incidence of and risk factors for sudden cardiac death in children with dilated cardiomyopathy: A report from the Pediatric Cardiomyopathy Registry. Journal of the American College of Cardiology. 2012;**59**(6):607-615

[91] Michels VV et al. Progression of familial and non-familial dilated cardiomyopathy: Long term follow up. Heart. 2003;**89**(7):757-761

[92] Miller WL et al. Troponin, B-type natriuretic peptides and outcomes in severe heart failure: Differences between ischemic and dilated cardiomyopathies. Clinical Cardiology. 2007;**30**(5):245-250

[93] Gulati A et al. Association of fibrosis with mortality and sudden cardiac death in patients with nonischemic dilated cardiomyopathy. JAMA. 2013;**309**(9):896-908

[94] Mahrholdt H et al. Delayed enhancement cardiovascular magnetic resonance assessment of non-ischaemic cardiomyopathies. European Heart Journal. 2005;**26**(15):1461-1474

[95] Pasotti M et al. Long-term outcome and risk stratification in dilated cardiolaminopathies. Journal of the American College of Cardiology. 2008;**52**(15):1250-1260

[96] Levy WC et al. The seattle heart failure model: Prediction of survival in heart failure. Circulation. 2006;**113**(11):1424-1433

[97] Priori SG et al. 2015 ESC Guidelines for the management of patients with ventricular arrhythmias and the prevention of sudden cardiac death: The Task Force for the Management of Patients with Ventricular Arrhythmias and the Prevention of Sudden Cardiac Death of the European Society of Cardiology (ESC). Endorsed by: Association for European Paediatric and Congenital Cardiology (AEPC). European Heart Journal. 2015;**36**(41):2793-2867

[98] Epstein AE et al. 2012 ACCF/AHA/HRS focused update incorporated into the ACCF/AHA/HRS 2008 guidelines for device-based therapy of cardiac rhythm abnormalities: A report of the American College of Cardiology Foundation/American Heart Association Task Force on Practice Guidelines and the Heart Rhythm Society. Journal of the American College of Cardiology. 2013;**61**(3):e6-e75

[99] Golwala H et al. Implantable cardioverter-defibrillator for nonischemic cardiomyopathy: An updated meta-analysis. Circulation. 2017;**135**(2):201-203

Chapter 5

# Modelling of Genetic Cardiac Diseases

*Chandra Prajapati and Katriina Aalto-Setälä*


## Abstract

Cardiac disease modeling is crucial to improve our understanding of the mechanism of various cardiac diseases and to discover new therapeutic approaches. Several modeling methods such as animal and computer simulations have been used to elucidate the cardiac diseases' mechanism and drug responses. However, each modeling technique has its own particular advantages and limitations. Human-based models would be particularly useful to investigate human cardiac diseases because humans and animals have differing cardiac physiologies and drug tolerability. In addition, the phenotype of cardiac diseases and response to therapeutic intervention differ not only between mutations but also among patients. Therefore, such diseases strongly demand the individualized/personalized strategies. Human-induced pluripotent stem cell-derived cardiomyocytes (hiPSC-CMs) offer the striking feature of retaining the same genetic information as donor, which guide us to investigate diseases and predict response to drug treatment individually. This feature of hiPSC-CMs is superior to the conventional in vitro modeling of cardiac diseases. Thus far, hiPSC-CMs have been successfully recapitulated many monogenic and also complex genetic cardiac diseases. hiPSC-CMs could be differentiated into different types of cardiomyocytes and non-cardiomyocyte cells, which empower us to understand cardiac chamber-specific arrhythmias such as atrial fibrillation and ventricular tachycardia.


**Keywords:** cardiac disease, modeling, hiPSC-CMs, drug

## 1. The importance of hiPSC-CMs

Cardiovascular diseases (CVDs) are the major causes of premature death and chronic disability worldwide [1]. Among CVD-related deaths, the occurrence of inherited lethal arrhythmias is the main reason for sudden cardiac death (SCD) in cardiac patients especially at young age [2]. Although many risk factors associated with SCD have been identified and understanding of pathogenesis of many cardiac diseases is progressing, the considerable number of cardiac patients still suffers SCD without warning, and we are still far from disease-specific treatment. Heterogeneous and multifactorial natures of genetic cardiac diseases are reasons for these complications. Furthermore, founder mutations causing cardiac disease have been reported in Finland [3], the Netherlands [4], and South Africa [5]. Not only disease phenotypes vary among different mutations, but also these vary among individuals carrying the same mutation. For example, long QT syndrome (LQTS) patients demonstrate a wide range of clinical phenotypes even among family members with the identical mutation [6]. Despite carrying the same gene variant resulting in cardiac disease, patients often demonstrate the wide spectrum of clinical outcomes ranging from the absence of distinct electrocardiogram (ECG) abnormalities and being lifelong asymptomatic to clear abnormalities in ECG (e.g., prolonged QT interval and arrhythmias) and premature SCD. In addition, SCD could also be the first manifestation of cardiac disease. These suggest that the type of genetic mutation cannot always be the sole factor that dictates the prognosis of disease and clinical phenotype in all individuals who carry it [7]. Thus, genetic cardiac diseases exhibit the incomplete penetrance and differ among genetic cardiac diseases. For example, Brugada syndrome (BrS) has a penetration range from 12.5 to 50%; mean penetrance of LQTS is ~40%, while overall penetrance of catecholaminergic polymorphic ventricular tachycardia (CPVT) is 78% [7]. Another convoluting factor that hinders the genotype-phenotype correlation is variable expressivity within one phenotype because some mutation carriers display all the phenotypic symptoms, whereas some only display part of mutation-specific phenotypes [8]. The clinical heterogeneity of genetic cardiac diseases suggests that ultimate disease severity (i.e., penetrance and expressivity) does not solely depend on one particular gene causing cardiac disease, but instead results from the combination of many modifying factors such as age, gender, and environmental and lifestyle factors, which either exacerbate or protect against disease [9]. In addition, patients carrying more than one disease-causing mutations (i.e., not polymorphisms) either in the same gene or different genes yield to more severe clinical disease including earlier onset of disease, early heart failure, and premature SCD [10]. Besides these, some of the cardiac diseases overlap their phenotypes with other cardiac diseases (**Figure 1**). For example, mutations in cardiac sodium ($Na^+$) channel gene, SCN5A, are associated with type 3 long QT (LQT3), BrS, cardiac conduction diseases, and sinus node dysfunction [11]. These incomplete penetrance, variable expressivity, and phenotypic overlap impede the complete understanding of diseases' mechanism as well as disease-specific treatment. Furthermore, the treatment therapies are mainly targeted for symptomatic patients to prevent and counteract the symptoms, but treatments in asymptomatic individuals are still of concern with variable opinions. Nevertheless, pharmacological therapies have been resulted in poor outcomes in the

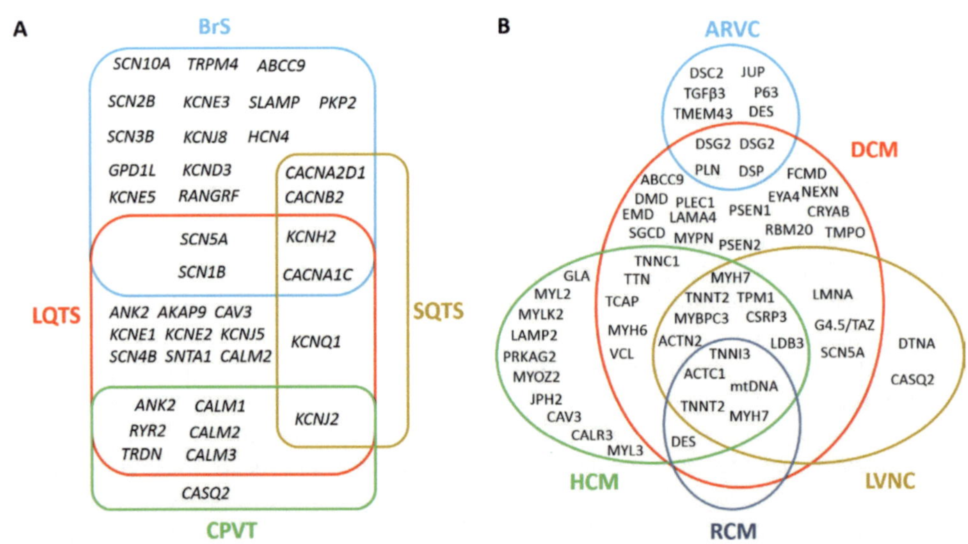


**Figure 1.**
*Heterogeneity of genetic cardiac diseases. (A) Overlapping genes causing channelopathies [27]. Brugada syndrome (BrS), long QT syndrome (LQTS), short QT syndrome (SQTS), catecholaminergic polymorphic ventricular tachycardia (CPVT) (ref). (B) Overlapping genes causing cardiomyopathies [72]. Arrhythmogenic right ventricular cardiomyopathy (ARVC), dilated cardiomyopathy (DCM), hypertrophic cardiomyopathy (HCM), restrictive cardiomyopathy (RCM), left ventricular non-compaction cardiomyopathy (LVNC).*

cardiac diseases [12]. So far, implantable cardioverter-defibrillator (ICD) is the only proven therapy for preventing detrimental consequences in cardiac patients with high risk of SCD [13]. However, ICD implantation is associated with its own complications and lower quality of life [14]. There are large groups of asymptomatic cardiac patients who do not have risk factors, which shift them into high-risk category as candidate for ICD implantation, but suffer SCD. Thus, the management for asymptomatic patients carrying pathogenic variant is the most challenging since SCD could be the first manifestation of disease [15, 16]. The clinical management of most cardiac diseases is suboptimal due to lack of comprehensive knowledge of mutations and possible mechanism involved. Thus, the mechanism of how mutation leads to modify the normal cardiac physiology and engender lethal arrhythmias should be deciphered so that the promising prevention and treatment could be established.

The prior cardiovascular research and drug screening have mostly been performed in animal models through knock-in/knock-out approaches. Although animal models have provided some fundamental information and led to many discoveries in genetic cardiac disease, physiological and pharmacological results cannot directly extrapolate from animals to humans because of some fundamental differences that exist between animal and human cardiac physiology [17]. For example, the resting heart rate of human is 75 bpm, while that of rat is 300 bpm, and the animal (mice and rats) can tolerate 6–400-fold higher concentration of some drugs compared to human [18]. The animal models become even worse when studying human cardiomyopathies due to mutations in contractile proteins, which are not highly expressed in mouse or rat. Therefore, it is more complicated to extrapolate physiological and pharmacological results from animal to human [17, 18]. Furthermore, most of cardiovascular drug screening and toxicology studies were performed in non-cardiac cell lines or animals, which do not accurately represent human CMs. Thus, considerable amount of cardiovascular drugs were withdrawn from market due to off-target effects [19]. Therefore, human tissues are required to study the human cardiac diseases and drug

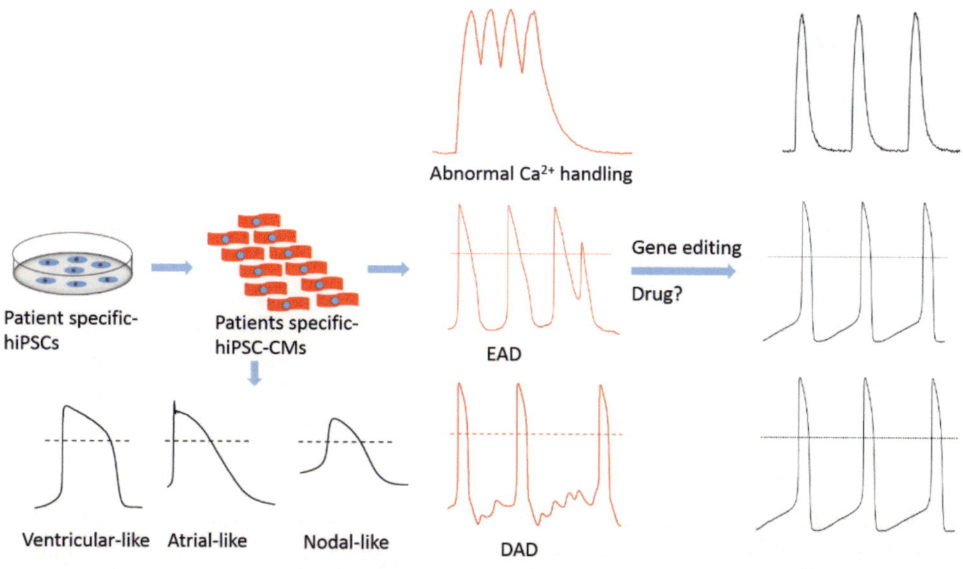


**Figure 2.**
*hiPSC-CM-based modeling of human genetic cardiac diseases. Human-induced pluripotent stem cells (hiPSCs) can be differentiated into hiPSC-derived cardiomyocytes (hiPSC-CMs). There are at least three subtypes of hiPSC-CMs, namely, ventricular-like, atrial-like, and nodal-like hiPSC-CMs. hiPSC-CMs derived from cardiac patients carrying genetic mutation recapitulate calcium and electrical abnormalities (early afterdepolarization (EAD) and delayed afterdepolarization (DAD)). Newly emerging gene editing techniques were able to mitigate these abnormalities in hiPSC-CMs.*

testing. However, the human sample exhibits some of the major challenges: there is limited supply of human cardiac biopsies, and it involves complex procedures and ethical issues. In addition, these cardiac biopsies are typically obtained from the end stage of cardiac diseases; hence it is not possible to understand the mechanism of cardiac diseases [20, 21]. These obstacles are mostly overcome by the groundbreaking discovery of reprogramming adult somatic cells into induced pluripotent stem cells (iPSCs) [22, 23] which can be differentiated into cardiomyocytes (CMs) (hiPSC-CMs) [24–26]. The main advantages of hiPSC-CMs are iPSCs can be generated at any period of a patient's life, they have unlimited supply, and these retain the same genetic information as the donor, i.e., hiPSC-CMs are patient specific (**Figure 2**). These are superior features of hiPSC-CMs to the conventional in vitro modeling of cardiac diseases. In addition, hiPSC-CMs can be cultured for several months, which enable us to study acute and chronic effect of mutation and drugs on CMs. Thus, hiPSC-CMs not only provide the platform to investigate the mutation-specific mechanism but also assist to anticipate drug response on an individual basis and guide us to personalized medicine in future.

## 2. Channelopathy phenotypes in hiPSC-CMs

Channelopathy cardiac diseases are caused by mutations in cardiac ion channels located in the cellular membrane or organelles. Mutations in ion channels result in misbalance of fine-tuning ion exchange during excitation-contraction coupling (ECC), which could lead to cardiac arrhythmias and SCD in the worst case. The main cardiac channelopathies are CPVT, LQTS, BrS, and short QT syndromes (SQTS) [27]. These cardiac channelopathies have been extensively studied using hiPSC-CMs and described below.

### 2.1 Catecholaminergic polymorphic ventricular tachycardia (CPVT)

CPVT is an inherited cardiac disease with the prevalence of about 1:5000/10,000. This disease is characterized by premature ventricular contraction and/or polymorphic ventricular tachycardia (VT) induced by adrenergic stimulation in response to emotional stress or physical exercise in structurally normal heart. Over 150 mutations in ryanodine receptor type 2 (*RYR2* gene) are responsible for ~ 55% of CPVT type 1 cases (CPVT1), and mutation in calsequestrin 2 (*CASQ2* gene) CPVT accounts for 3–5% CPVT type 2 (CPVT2) cases [28, 29]. In addition, mutations in calmodulin (CALM1) genes and in triadin (TRDN) have been reported causing CPVT. *RYR2*, *CASQ2*, CALM1, and TRDN are involved in ECC, and mutation in any of these genes results in elevated intracellular $Ca^{2+}$, which leads to abnormal $Ca^{2+}$ handling and arrhythmias [28, 29]. In consistency with clinical phenotype, many hiPSC-CM model had demonstrated the exacerbation of electrophysiological and $Ca^{2+}$ handling abnormalities upon adrenergic stimulation [26, 30–32]. Furthermore, Zhang and colleagues had modeled hiPSC-CMs harboring CPVT1-associated F2483I mutation in *RYR2* gene and demonstrated that CPVT1 hiPSC-CMs had longer and wandering $Ca^{2+}$ sparks and smaller sarcoplasmic reticulum $Ca^{2+}$ content [32]. Later on, the same group corrected this mutation using clustered regularly interspaced short palindromic repeats/Cas9 (CRISPR/Cas9) gene editing technique and showed that this mutation is causative rather than associative to the disease [33]. hiPSC-CM model for CPVT has also been used in studying the efficacy of various drugs. Previously we had directly compared the clinical results from CPVT1 patients with dantrolene medication, and the clinical response of dantrolene was similar as in hiPSC-CMs from the same patients; dantrolene abolished or markedly reduced arrhythmias in patients and their hiPSC-CMs with certain mutation in *RYR2*, while it did not have any clinical effect with hiPSC-CMs or with other *RYR2* mutations [31]. Furthermore, an antiarrhythmic drug, flecainide, used to treat CPVT1 patients [34] was able to reduce the $Ca^{2+}$ irregularities under adrenergic stimulation in CPVT1 hiPSC-CMs [30, 35]. CPVT2 patients harboring homozygous CASQ2-G112 + 5X mutation in *CASQ2* gene showed the rapid polymorphic VT under exercise stress test [36]. Adult rat ventricular myocytes were studied to understand the effect of *CASQ2* mutation in ECC, demonstrating that mutated CMs exhibited spontaneous extrasystolic $Ca^{2+}$ elevations and delayed afterdepolarization (DADs) upon adrenergic stimulation [36]. Later, hiPSC-CM model harboring CASQ2-G112 + 5X mutation emulated these phenotypic features of disease, and AAV9-based gene delivery effectively prevents the development of adrenergic-induced DADs and triggered arrhythmias in CPVT2 hiPSC-CMs [37].

### 2.2 LQT type 1 (LQT1)

LQT type 1 (LQT1) is caused by loss-of-function mutation in *KCNQ1* gene encoding α subunit of potassium ($K^+$) channel mediating slow delayed rectifier $K^+$ current ($I_{Ks}$). LQT1 is responsible for 30–35% of all LQTS cases [38]. LQT1 is characterized by prolongation of QT interval in ECG, which could lead to SCD due to VT, typically torsades de pointes [39]. hiPSC-CMs derived from LQT1 patients faithfully recapitulated the clinical hallmark by showing prolonged action potential duration (APD) which is analogous to QT duration in ECG, and reduced $I_{Ks}$ current densities are held responsible for abnormal repolarization [40–42]. ML277, an $I_{Ks}$ activator, increased the $I_{Ks}$ amplitude by enhancing the activation of $I_{Ks}$, thus resulting in shortening of APD in LQT1 hiPSC-CMs [40]. In addition, adrenergic stimulation in LQT1 hiPSC-CMs induced the early afterdepolarization (EAD) [42], which is similar to arrhythmias triggered in LQT1 patients by exercise or emotional stress [39]. Clinically, β-blockers were effective in minimizing the risk of cardiac events in LQT1 patients [43]. Similar antiarrhythmic effect of β-blockers has been observed in LQT1 hiPSC-CMs [42]. Furthermore, hypokalemia is the electrolyte disturbance caused by lower $K^+$ level in blood serum, which aggravates the QT prolongation and facilitates the development of hypokalemia-induced torsades de pointes in LQT1 patients [39, 44]. We successfully developed and mimicked these disease phenotypes in LQT1 hiPSC-CMs carrying G589D or IVS7-2A > G mutation in *KCNQ1* gene. Additionally, lowering the extracellular $K^+$ concentration prolonged APDs and induced the formation of EADs in LQT1 hiPSC-CMs [45]. Both G589D- and IVS7-2A > G-specific LQT1 hiPSC-CMs displayed longer APD and higher $Ca^{2+}$ abnormalities in baseline; G589D hiPSC-CMs demonstrated prolonged contraction, while IVS7-2A > G hiPSC-CMs showed impaired relaxation [46] observed in our video image-based software analysis [47].

### 2.3 LQT type 2 (LQT2)

LQT type 2 (LQT2) is an LQTS subtype, which is caused by loss-of-function mutations in *KCNH2* gene also known as human ether-a-go-go-related gene (*hERG*) encoding $K^+$ channel mediating rapid delayed rectifier K current ($I_{Kr}$). LQT2 is responsible for approximately 25–30% of all LQTS cases [38]. Similar to LQT1, LQT2 patients also exhibit the prolongation of QT interval and torsades de pointes. As in LQT1 hiPSC-CM model, LQT2 hiPSC-CMs also recapitulated clinical phenotypes by displaying longer APD resulted from reduced $I_{Kr}$ current densities and enhanced EAD following the adrenergic stimulation [48–50]. Our early study of LQT2 hiPSC-CMs carrying R176W mutation in *KCNH2* gene demonstrated the reduced $I_{Kr}$ current densities, prolonged repolarization, and increased arrhythmogenicity although the donor is an asymptomatic carrier [50]. These results are in parallel with clinical findings that LQT2 patients usually display symptoms when heart rate is slow. In addition, this report illustrated that electrophysiological abnormalities can be detected in hiPSC-CMs, although iPSCs are derived from asymptomatic carriers of *KCNH2* mutations. The application of $I_{Kr}$ blockers (E4031 and sotalol) further prolonged the APD resulting in EADs, whereas $Ca^{2+}$ channel blocker (nifedipine), $I_{K,ATP}$ channel opener (pinacidil and nicorandil), and $I_{Kr}$ channel enhancer (PD-118057) reduced the APD and thus mitigated the formation of EAD in LQT2 hiPSC-CMs [48, 49]. Several novel pharmacological strategies including ICA-105574 (potent $I_{Kr}$ activator) [51], chaperone modulator N-[N-(N-acetyl-L-leucyl)-L-leucyl]-L-norleucine (ALLN) [52], LUF7346 (hERG allosteric modulators) [53], as well as application of allele-specific RNA interference approach [54] have been attempts to rescue the LQT phenotype in LQT2 hiPSC-CMs. Correcting the mutation associated with LQT2 not only confirmed that mutation caused $I_{Kr}$ reduction and APD prolongation but also suggested that trafficking defect as the pathological mechanism is responsible for the electrophysiological phenotype in LQT2 [51, 55].

## 2.4 LQT type 3 (LQT3)

LQT type 3 (LQT3) is caused by gain-of-function mutations in SCN5A encoding α subunit of cardiac $Na^+$ channels [56]. The gain-of-function SCN5A mutation results in augmented late or persistent $Na^+$ current ($I_{NaL}$), which leads to prolongation of QT interval in ECG and proarrhythmia. LQT3 is the third most common LQTS accounting for 5–10% of all LQTS cases [56]. LQT3 patients exhibit longer QT duration at slower heart rate, thus LQT3 patients are at higher risk for cardiac events during rest or sleep [57]. LQT3 patients harboring V1763 M mutation in *SCN5A* [58] R1644H mutation in *SCN5A* [59] or F1473C mutation in *SCN5A* and a polymorphism (K897 T) in *KCNH2* [60] had prolonged QT interval, and in vitro models using hiPSC-CMs derived from all those LQT3 patients demonstrated prolonged APD resulting in the larger $I_{Na,L}$ and altered biophysical properties of $Na^+$ channels [58–60]. Mexiletine, a $Na^+$ channel inhibitor commonly used in LQT3 therapy, lowered the $I_{Na,L}$ and thereby rescued the APD prolongation phenotype [58, 59] and suppressed the occurrence of EAD [59] and also corrected the altered $Na^+$ channel inactivation [60]. Incorporating the biophysics of $Na^+$ channel and pharmacological analysis illustrated that the improper functioning of $Na^+$ channel was responsible for LQT3 phenotypes rather than *KCNH2* polymorphism [60]. In addition to LQT3, mutation in *SCN5A* gene can cause BrS, and mixed phenotypes are often seen, which is also known as the "overlap syndrome." Loss in function of $Na^+$ channel is often seen in BrS. Liang and co-workers had generated hiPSCs from two BrS patients, one with double missense mutation (R620H and R811H) in *SCN5A* gene (BrS(p1)) and another with one-base pair deletion mutation in the *SCN5A* gene (BrS(p2)), and showed that BrS hiPSC-CMs derived from both patients had reduced $Na^+$ current and increased triggered activity and abnormal $Ca^{2+}$ handling [61]. These phenotypes were alleviated by correcting the mutation by CRISPR/Cas9 in hiPSCs derived from BrS (p2) [61]. Importantly, only BrS hiPSC-CMs harboring BrS-associated SCN5A-1795insD mutation displayed reduced $Na^+$ current and upstroke velocity, but not with three sets of hiPSC-CMs derived from BrS patients who tested negative for mutations in the known BrS-associated genes suggesting the $Na^+$ channel dysfunction may not be prerequisite for BrS [62]. In another study, $Na^+$ current and upstroke velocity were reduced, but not the voltage-dependent inactivation in BrS hiPSC-CMs carrying the mutations R1638X and W156X [63].

## 2.5 LQT type 7 (LQT7) or Andersen-Tawil syndrome (ATS)

LQT type 7 (LQT7) or Andersen-Tawil syndrome (ATS) is a rare inherited cardiac disease associated with mutation in *KCNJ2* gene (ATS type 1) encoding inward rectifying $K^+$ channel (Kir2.1) and accounts for ~70% of all ATS cases. However, the genetic cause of the remaining 30% of ATS (ATS type 2) remains unknown. In ATS patients, QT interval prolongation is not common, but prominent U wave and QU interval in ECG could be hallmarks of ATS, and they experienced cardiac arrhythmias including non-sustained VT and torsade de pointes [64]. Kuroda and co-workers generated hiPSCs from ATS patients carrying R218W, R67W, and R218Q mutations in *KCNJ2* gene and showed strong arrhythmic events and higher incidence of irregular $Ca^{2+}$ handling in ATS hiPSC-CMs, but flecainide and KB-R7943 (a reverse-mode $Na^+/Ca^{2+}$ exchanger inhibitor) were able to suppress those events [65].

### 2.6 LQT type 8 (LQT8) or Timothy syndrome (TS)

2.6 LQT type 8 (LQT8) or Timothy syndrome (TS) is a very rare genetic cardiac disease which results from mutation in *CACNA1C* gene encoding $Ca^{2+}$ channel ($Ca_V$1.2). LQT8 is the most severe type of LQTS, which is characterized by markedly prolonged QT interval, severe ventricular arrhythmia, and multiorgan dysfunction [66]. hiPSC-CMs derived from TS patients recapitulated the disease phenotypes, but roscovitine rescued those abnormalities such as altered $Ca^{2+}$ channel inactivation, prolonged APD, higher incidences of arrhythmias, and abnormal $Ca^{2+}$ handling [67].

### 2.7 Short QT (SQT)

SQT is a rare inherited cardiac disease characterized by QT internal shortening, which is in contrast to QT prolongation observed in LQTS. SQT is associated with mutations in genes associated with $K^+$ channel or $Ca^{2+}$ channels [68]. The prevalence of SQT is between 0.02–0.1% and 0.05% in adults and children, respectively [69]. Recently El-Battrawy and co-workers had generated hiPSCs from SQT type 1 patients carrying a mutation (N588K) in *KCNH2*, and hiPSC-CMs mimicked the clinical phenotype of SQT by showing a shortened APD as a result of increased $I_{Kr}$ current densities [70]. In addition, SQT hiPSC-CMs exhibited abnormal $Ca^{2+}$ transients and rhythmic activities, which are enhanced by carbachol, but quinidine alleviated those carbachol-induced arrhythmias and prolonged the APD [70].

## 3. Cardiomyopathy phenotypes in hiPSC-CMs

Cardiomyopathies are diseases of cardiac muscle and associated with structural and/or functional abnormalities. The most common genetic cardiomyopathies are hypertrophic cardiomyopathy (HCM), dilated cardiomyopathy (DCM), and arrhythmogenic right ventricular cardiomyopathy/dysplasia (ARVC/D). These genetic cardiomyopathies have been also extensively studied using hiPSC-CMs [71, 72].

### 3.1 Hypertrophic cardiomyopathy (HCM)

HCM is one of the most common genetic cardiac diseases with an estimate prevalence of 1 in 500. HCM is characterized by unexplained symmetrical or asymmetrical left ventricular hypertrophy. Mutations in sarcomeric proteins account for ~60% of all HCM cases including mutation in β-myosin heavy chain (MYH7), cardiac myosin-binding protein C (MYBPC3), cardiac troponin I (cTnI), cardiac troponin T (cTnT), and tropomyosin (TPM1) [73]. Hypertrophy of myocytes and disarray of sarcomere are the histological hallmarks of HCM seen in cardiac biopsies from HCM patients [74], and these histological phenotypes are also observed in hiPSC-CM model of HCM [25, 75–77]. In addition, HCM hiPSC-CMs also demonstrated other hallmarks of HCM such as nuclear translocation of nuclear factor of activated T cells (NFAT) [75–77], elevation of β-myosin/α-myosin ratio, and calcineurin activation [75]. Furthermore, isolated CMs from HCM patients displayed the prolonged APDs, increased $Ca^{2+}$ current densities, reduced transient outward $K^+$ current densities, abnormal $Ca^{2+}$ handling, and increased frequency of arrhythmias [21]. These electrophysiological and $Ca^{2+}$ transient irregularity phenotypes have been faithfully recapitulated in HCM hiPSC-CMs [25, 75, 76, 78]. When HCM tissues carrying a mutation in *MYBPC3* gene were compared with donor heart sample, no specific truncated MyBP-C peptides were detected, but the overall level of MyBP-C in myofibrils was significantly reduced [79]. Similar haploinsufficiency results were also shown in HCM hiPSC-CMs with mutation in *MYBPC3* gene [25, 80], and gene replacement in HCM hiPSC-CMs partially improves the haploinsufficiency and reduces cellular hypertrophy [80]. Similar to higher myofilament $Ca^{2+}$ sensitivity observed in isolated cardiac biopsies from HCM with E99K mutation in cardiac actin [81], in vitro model of HCM hiPSC-CMs carrying E99K mutation in cardiac actin demonstrated significantly stronger contraction and increased arrhythmogenic events [82] Furthermore, a study in HCM mice harboring I79N mutation in cTnT resulted in increased cardiac contractility, altered $Ca^{2+}$ transients, and remodeling of action potential [83]. These phenotypes were faithfully recapitulated by HCM hiPSC-CMs carrying the same I79N mutation in cTnT [84]. These hypercontractility and increased arrhythmogenicity phenotypes were reversed in HCM hiPSC-CMs when the E99K mutation in cardiac actin [82] and I79N mutation in cTnT [84] were corrected using CRISPR/Cas9 gene editing technique. Recently, we have shown that HCM hiPSC-CMs carrying *TPM1-Asp175Asn* mutation exhibited VT type of arrhythmias [78], and this observation is in line with earlier clinical observation of HCM patients with *TPM1-Asp175Asn* mutation being at increased risk of fatal arrhythmias [85]. Currently, there is no specific pharmacological therapy for HCM patients, and drugs are prescribed mainly based on symptoms and personal history. However, drug therapy has also resulted in poor outcomes in HCM patients [12]. We reported the similar poor antiarrhythmic efficiency of β-blocker in preventing lethal arrhythmias in HCM hiPSC-CMs [78]. In another HCM report, several environmental factors were investigated with hiPSC-CMs to study their effect on disease progression [77]. They found that endothelin (ET)-1 was able to induce HCM phenotypes such as cellular hypertrophy and myofibrillar disarray in hiPSC-CMs, which are inhibited by ET receptor type A blocker [77]. HCM patients exhibited defects in mitochondrial functions and ultrastructure and abnormal energy metabolism [74]. These structural and functional phenotypes were recapitulated in hiPSC-CMs carrying m.2336 T > C mutation in mitochondrial genome causing HCM [86]. They reported that HCM hiPSC-CMs expressed reduced levels of mitochondrial proteins, ATP/ADP ratio, and mitochondrial membrane potential [86].

### 3.2 Dilated cardiomyopathy (DCM)

DCM is a myocardial disease characterized by ventricular chamber enlargement and systolic dysfunction and progressive heart failure without significant change in ventricular wall thickness. Mutations in >30 genes encoding proteins of cytoskeleton, sarcomere, and nuclear lamina are found in 30–35% of DCM patients [87]. DCM patients with mutations in *RBM20*, encoding RNA binding motif protein 20 (RBM20), have an early onset of disease phenotype [88]. Isolated CMs from DCM patients carrying mutation in RBM20 displayed elongated and thinner sarcomere structure [88], and such disorganized sarcomeric structure phenotypes were recapitulated in DCM hiPSC-CMs carrying mutation in RBM20 [89, 90]. RBM20 is the main regulator of the heart-specific titin splicing, and N2BA isoform is predominantly expressed in CMs from DCM patient carrying mutation in the *RBM20* gene [91]. In vitro model of RBM20 hiPSC-CMs successfully mirrored the altered titin isoform expression (titin isoform switch) [89, 90]. Furthermore, RBM20 hiPSC-CMs showed delayed $Ca^{2+}$ extrusion and reuptake and more $Ca^{2+}$ being released during each ECC, which resulted into deficient muscle contraction, the hallmark of cardiac dysfunction of DCM patients [89, 90]. In addition, a three-dimensional engineered heart muscle generated from RBM20 hiPSC-CMs showed an impaired force of contraction, and passive stress was decreased in response to stepwise increase in strain, suggesting higher viscoelasticity caused by mutation in *RBM20* [89]. Besides HCM, mutation in cTnT also caused DCM and resulted in shifts in $Ca^{2+}$ sensitivity and force of contraction [92]. Sun and co-workers generated iPSCs from DCM patients carrying R173W mutation in cTnT and reported that DCM hiPSC-CMs exhibited altered $Ca^{2+}$ handling, decreased contractility, and abnormal sarcomeric α–actinin distribution [93]. DCM patients with lamin A/C (LMNA) mutations show a highly variable phenotype. Cardiac biopsies from DCM patients harboring LMNA mutations exhibit reduced LMNA in nuclei with nuclear membrane damage such as focal disruption and nuclear pore clustering [94]. Nonsense mutation (R225X) in exon 4 of the LMNA gene causing DCM was associated with accelerated nuclear senescence and apoptosis of DCM hiPSC-CMs under electrical stimulation [95]. In another in vitro modeling of DCM, harboring A285V mutation in desmin (*DES*) using hiPSC-CMs displayed the pathogenic phenotypes of DCM such as diffuse abnormal DES aggregation, poor co-localization of DES with cTnT, and Z-disk streaming with accumulation of granulofilamentous materials or pleomorphic dense structures adjacent to the Z-disk or between the myofibrils [96]. DCM patients harboring R14del mutation in phospholamban (PLN) result in ventricular dilation, contractile dysfunction, and episodic ventricular arrhythmias [97]. Similarly, hiPSC-CMs carrying R14del mutation in PLN induced the $Ca^{2+}$ handling abnormalities, irregular electrical activity, and abnormal intracellular distribution of PLN in DCM hiPSC-CMs [98]. These PLN R14del-associated disease phenotypes were mitigated upon correction of PLN R14del mutation by transcription activator-like effector nuclease (TALENs) gene editing technique [98]. Furthermore, genetic correction of PLN R14del mutation by TALENs improved the force development and restored the contractile function in three-dimensional human engineered cardiac tissue derived from R14del-iPSCs [99].

### 3.3 Arrhythmogenic right ventricular cardiomyopathy (ARVC)

ARVC is rare genetic cardiac disease with the prevalence ranging from 1:000 to 1:5000 worldwide. The histopathological hallmark of ARVC is the substitution of the cardiac myocytes with fibro-fatty deposits, particularly within the free wall of the right ventricle. The consequent results from the disruption of normal myocardial architecture can lead to right ventricular dysfunction, life-threatening arrhythmias, and SCD [100]. ARVC is caused by mutations in genes encoding desmosomal proteins such as plakoglobin (JUP), desmoplakin (DSP), plakophilin-2 (PKP2), desmoglein-2 (DSG2), and desmocollin-2 (DSC2) [100]. Similar to immunohistological results from the biopsy sample from ARVC patients [101], ARVC hiPSC-CMs harboring a plakophilin 2 (PKP2) gene mutation mimicked the reduced *PKP2* immunosignal [102, 103]. In addition, clusters of lipid droplets accumulating within the cytoplasm were identified in ARVC-hiPSC-CMs associated with structural distortion of desmosomes [103]. Another study showed that induction of adult-like metabolic energetics from an embryonic/glycolytic state and abnormal peroxisome proliferator-activated receptor gamma (PPARγ) activation underlie the pathogenesis of ARVC [104]. It has been observed that male ARVC patients develop earlier and more severe phenotype than female ARVC patients [105]. To understand whether sex hormones in serum may contribute to the major arrhythmic cardiovascular events in ARVC, Akdis and co-workers combined a clinical study and in vitro hiPSC-CM model and showed that increased levels of testosterone accelerate ARVC pathologies, while premenopausal female estradiol levels slow down exaggerated apoptosis and lipid accumulation in ARVC hiPSC-CMs [106].

## 4. Limitations and future prospective

The reprogramming of somatic cells into pluripotent stems cells and subsequent differentiation into specific cell types is a newly emerging technique and is certainly not free from limitation.

One of the most questionable issues of hiPSC-CMs is their maturity. Despite expressing relevant ion channels [107] and structural genes [25, 26, 75, 76, 89, 108], hiPSC-CMs lack t-tubules and exhibit lower expression of Kir2.1 and weaker contractility; thus they do not fully resemble adult CMs. In order to improve the maturity of hiPSC-CMs and consequently upgrade the functionality of hiPSC-CMs, various techniques have been investigated in different groups. Three-dimensional construction of engineered heart tissue is a rapidly growing technique for structural and functional maturations of hiPSC-CMs [109], which resulted in higher $Na^+$ current density and upstroke velocity [110], and enhances the metabolic maturation [111] comparable to adult CMs. Furthermore, Shadrin and co-workers introduced the "Cardiopatch" platform for three-dimensional culture and maturation of hiPSC-CMs; this platform produces robust electromechanical coupling, consistent H-zone and I bands, and evidence of t-tubules and M-bands [112].

Another issue of hiPSC-CMs is the purity of differentiated CMs. The CMs differentiated from hiPSCs yield in heterogeneous population of CMs. There are at least three subtypes of CMs such as ventricular, atrial, and nodal CMs; among them the majority (~70%) of CMs are ventricular-like, and only a minority of CMs are atrial-like (~20%) and nodal-like (~10%) [40, 58, 93, 107]. Although many molecular and functional characteristics are shared among these CMs subtypes, they also exhibit their own unique features. For example, ventricular CMs have prominent plateau phase (phase 2) in action potential profile, atrial CMs exclusively exhibit $I_{Kur}$ channels, and nodal CMs lack strong upstroke velocity [113]. Most of the published methods of differentiation protocol yield in a lower amount of atrial-like and nodal-like CMs [40, 58, 93, 107], but sufficient numbers of subtype-specific CMs are needed to understand the subtype-related disease mechanism and development of specific therapeutic approaches. Atrial fibrillation (AF) is one of the most common cardiac arrhythmias; however, current antiarrhythmic drugs for treatment of AF are not atrial-specific and could cause unacceptable ventricular events [114]. Thus, sufficient supply of atrial CMs is crucial for investigating the AF cellular mechanism. hiPSCs have been differentiated into high-purity atrial-specific CMs by using retinoic acid signaling at the mesoderm stage of development [115]. These patient-specific atrial CMs allow us to investigate in detail mechanisms of AF and to develop atrial-specific therapeutic drugs. Furthermore, sinoatrial node (SAN) dysfunction can manifest bradycardia and asystolic pauses, but its pathophysiology is not completely understood [116]. SAN pacemaker cells from hiPSCs would facilitate the study of the disease mechanism and provide a cell source for developing a biological pacemaker. Protze and co-workers had reported the transgene-independent method for the generation of pacemaker cells (nodal-like CMs) from human pluripotent stem cells by stage-specific manipulation of developmental signaling pathways [117]. Besides CMs, the heart also consists of many other cell types such as fibroblast, endothelial and vascular smooth muscle cells, and also extracellular matrix. Importantly, the origin of cardiac diseases may not always exclusively originate from CMs, but might involve non-CMs. Thus, incorporating the fibroblasts [118], endothelial cells [119], and vascular smooth muscle cells [120] into CMs from the same hiPSCs could offer new insight of disease mechanism.

The establishment of appropriate control is another challenge in disease modeling using hiPSC-CMs. It is generally argued/suggested that when comparing the results between control and mutated hiPSC-CMs, both should have the same genetic background. This objective is achieved in somehow by using healthy family members as control [58, 93]. However, only ~50% of genome is shared between siblings, and phenotypic difference could result from DNA variants in the rest of genome besides disease-associated mutation [121]. Mutated genes can be corrected with the help of newly growing gene editing technology such as TALENs [98] and CRISPR/Cas9 [33, 51, 84], thus establishing the so-called isogenic lines. This isogenic line would be the most appropriate control for comparison as it differs only in the presence and absence of mutation. Therefore, advance genome engineering will not only provide more reliable control lines but also guide us to understand how mutation modifies the normal functioning of cells. However, for diseased CMs without known mutation, healthy family members or otherwise controls are still the best.

## 5. Conclusion

While animal models fail to recapitulate human cardiac disease phenotype properly, hiPSC-CMs have been successful in recapitulating crucial phenotypes of many genetic cardiac diseases in terms of morphology, contractility, $Ca^{2+}$ handling, ion channel biophysics, cell signaling, and metabolism. Most strikingly, hiPSC-CMs provide the patient-specific platform to study the disease mechanism and drug response individually, which the traditional disease modeling technique would never offer. In addition, cardiac subtype-specific arrhythmias and drug screening could be performed with the help of unlimited supply of hiPSC-CMs; thus chamber-specific treatment modalities could be identified. Certainly, by improving the current weaknesses of hiPSC-CMs and incorporating with new gene editing techniques, complex cardiac disease mechanism could be deciphered, and novel effective treatment therapies could be identified to improve the life of cardiac patients.

## Acknowledgements

We would like to thank funders for our research group: Tekes–Finnish Funding Agency for Innovation, Academy of Finland, and Finnish Cardiovascular Research Foundation.

## Conflict of interest

No conflict of interest.

## Abbreviations

| | |
|---|---|
| AF | atrial fibrillation |
| ARVC/D | arrhythmogenic right ventricular cardiomyopathy/dysplasia |
| APD | action potential duration |
| ATS | Andersen-Tawil syndrome |

| | |
|---|---|
| BrS | Brugada syndrome |
| $Ca^{2+}$ | calcium ion |
| CPVT | catecholaminergic polymorphic ventricular tachycardia |
| CRISPR | clustered regularly interspaced short palindromic repeats |
| cTnT | cardiac troponin T |
| CVDs | cardiovascular diseases |
| DADs | delayed afterdepolarization |
| DCM | dilated cardiomyopathy |
| DSC2 | desmocollin-2 |
| DSG2 | desmoglein-2 |
| DSP | desmoplakin |
| EAD | early afterdepolarization |
| ECC | excitation-contraction coupling |
| ECG | electrocardiogram |
| ET | endothelin |
| hiPSC-CMs | human-induced pluripotent stem cell-derived cardiomyocytes |
| ICD | implantable cardioverter-defibrillator |
| iPSCs | induced pluripotent stem cells |
| $K^+$ | potassium ion |
| LMNA | lamin A/C |
| LQTS | long QT syndromes |
| MYBPC3 | cardiac myosin-binding protein C |
| MYH7 | myosin heavy chain |
| $Na^+$ | sodium ion |
| PKP2 | plakophilin-2 |
| PLN | phospholamban |
| SAN | sinoatrial node |
| SCD | sudden cardiac death |
| SQTS | short QT syndromes |
| TALENs | transcription activator-like effector nucleases |
| TS | Timothy syndrome |
| VT | ventricular tachycardia |

## Author details

Chandra Prajapati[1] and Katriina Aalto-Setälä[1,2]*

1 Faculty of Medicine and Life Technology, BioMediTech, University of Tampere, Tampere, Finland

2 Heart Hospital, Tampere University Hospital, Tampere, Finland

*Address all correspondence to: katriina.aalto-setala@uta.fi

## References

[1] Roth GA, Johnson C, Abajobir A, Abd-Allah F, Abera SF, Abyu G, et al. Global, regional, and national burden of cardiovascular diseases for 10 causes, 1990 to 2015. Journal of the American College of Cardiology. 2017;**70**(1):1-25

[2] Meyer L, Stubbs B, Fahrenbruch C, Maeda C, Harmon K, Eisenberg M, et al. Incidence, causes, and survival trends from cardiovascular-related sudden cardiac arrest in children and young adults 0 to 35 years of age: A 30-year review. Circulation. 2012;**126**(11):1363-1372

[3] Jääskelainen P, Helio T, Aalto-Setala K, Kaartinen M, Ilveskoski E, Hamalainen L, et al. Two founder mutations in the alpha-tropomyosin and the cardiac myosin-binding protein C genes are common causes of hypertrophic cardiomyopathy in the Finnish population. Annals of Medicine. 2013;**45**(1):85-90

[4] Christiaans I, Nannenberg EA, Dooijes D, Jongbloed RJE, Michels M, Postema PG, et al. Founder mutations in hypertrophic cardiomyopathy patients in the Netherlands. Netherlands heart journal: Monthly journal of the Netherlands Society of Cardiology and the Netherlands Heart Foundation. 2010;**18**(5):248-254

[5] Brink PA, Crotti L, Corfield V, Goosen A, Durrheim G, Hedley P, et al. Phenotypic variability and unusual clinical severity of congenital long-QT syndrome in a founder population. Circulation. 2005;**112**(17):2602-2610

[6] Giudicessi JR, Ackerman MJ. Genotype- and phenotype-guided management of congenital long QT syndrome. Current Problems in Cardiology. 2013;**38**(10):417-455

[7] Giudicessi JR, Ackerman MJ. Determinants of incomplete penetrance and variable expressivity in heritable cardiac arrhythmia syndromes. Translational Research. 2013;**161**:1-14

[8] Shinozawa T, Nakamura K, Shoji M, Morita M, Kimura M, Furukawa H, et al. Recapitulation of clinical individual susceptibility to drug-induced QT prolongation in healthy subjects using iPSC-derived cardiomyocytes. Stem Cell Reports. 2017;**8**(2):226-234

[9] Coll M, Pérez-Serra A, Mates J, del Olmo B, Puigmulé M, Fernandez-Falgueras A, et al. Incomplete penetrance and variable expressivity: Hallmarks in channelopathies associated with sudden cardiac death. Biology (Basel) [Internet]. 2017;7(1):3. Available from: http://www.mdpi.com/2079-7737/7/1/3

[10] Kelly M, Semsarian C, Cirino AL, Ho CY, Ashley EA. Multiple mutations in genetic cardiovascular disease: A marker of disease severity? Circulation: Cardiovascular Genetics [Internet]. 2009;**2**(2):182-190. Available from: http://www.ncbi.nlm.nih.gov/pubmed/20031583

[11] Veltmann C, Barajas-Martinez H, Wolpert C, Borggrefe M, Schimpf R, Pfeiffer R, et al. Further insights in the most common SCN5A mutation causing overlapping phenotype of long QT syndrome, Brugada syndrome, and conduction defect. Journal of the American Heart Association. 2016;**5**(7)

[12] Spoladore R, Maron MS, D'Amato R, Camici PG, Olivotto I. Pharmacological treatment options for hypertrophic cardiomyopathy: High time for evidence. European Heart Journal. 2012;**33**:1724-1733

[13] McAnulty J, Halperin B, Kron J, Larsen G, Raitt M, Swenson R, et al. A comparison of antiarrhythmic-drug therapy with implantable

defibrillators in patients resuscitated from near-fatal ventricular arrhythmias. New England Journal of Medicine. 1997;**337**(22):1576-1583

[14] Olde Nordkamp LRA, Postema PG, Knops RE, Van Dijk N, Limpens J, Wilde AAM, et al. Implantable cardioverter-defibrillator harm in young patients with inherited arrhythmia syndromes: A systematic review and meta-analysis of inappropriate shocks and complications. Heart Rhythm. 2016;**13**(2):443-454

[15] Suzuki H, Hoshina S, Ozawa J, Sato A, Minamino T, Aizawa Y, et al. Short QT syndrome in a boy diagnosed on screening for heart disease. Pediatrics International. 2014;**56**(5):774-776

[16] Giustetto C, Schimpf R, Mazzanti A, Scrocco C, Maury P, Anttonen O, et al. Long-term follow-up of patients with short QT syndrome. Journal of the American College of Cardiology. 2011;**58**(6):587-595

[17] Farraj AK, Hazari MS, Cascio WE. The utility of the small rodent electrocardiogram in toxicology. Toxicological Sciences. 2011;**121**:11-30

[18] Jung G, Bernstein D. hiPSC modeling of inherited cardiomyopathies. Current Treatment Options in Cardiovascular Medicine [Internet]. 2014;**16**(7):320. Available from: http://www.ncbi.nlm.nih.gov/pubmed/24838688%0Ahttp://www.pubmedcentral.nih.gov/articlerender.fcgi?artid=PMC4096486

[19] Munos B. Lessons from 60 years of pharmaceutical innovation. Nature Reviews. Drug Discovery. 2009;**8**:959-968

[20] Barajas-Martínez H, Hu D, Goodrow RJ, Joyce F, Antzelevitch C. Electrophysiologic characteristics and pharmacologic response of human cardiomyocytes isolated from a patient with hypertrophic cardiomyopathy. PACE—Pacing and Clinical Electrophysiology. 2013;**36**(12):1512-1515

[21] Coppini R, Ferrantini C, Yao L, Fan P, Del Lungo M, Stillitano F, et al. Late sodium current inhibition reverses electromechanical dysfunction in human hypertrophic cardiomyopathy. Circulation. 2013;**127**(5):575-584

[22] Takahashi K, Tanabe K, Ohnuki M, Narita M, Ichisaka T, Tomoda K, et al. Induction of pluripotent stem cells from adult human fibroblasts by defined factors. Cell. 2007;**131**(5):861-872

[23] Yu J, Vodyanik MA, Smuga-Otto K, Antosiewicz-Bourget J, Frane JL, Tian S, et al. Induced pluripotent stem cell lines derived from human somatic cells. Science (80-). 2007;**318**(5858):1917-1920

[24] Kujala K, Paavola J, Lahti A, Larsson K, Pekkanen-Mattila M, Viitasalo M, et al. Cell model of catecholaminergic polymorphic ventricular tachycardia reveals early and delayed afterdepolarizations. PLoS One. 2012;7(9):e44660

[25] Ojala M, Prajapati C, Pölönen R-P, Rajala K, Pekkanen-Mattila M, Rasku J, et al. Mutation-specific phenotypes in hiPSC-derived cardiomyocytes carrying either myosin-binding protein C or α-tropomyosin mutation for hypertrophic cardiomyopathy. Stem Cells International. 2016. Article ID: 1684792

[26] Novak A, Barad L, Lorber A, Gherghiceanu M, Reiter I, Eisen B, et al. Functional abnormalities in iPSC-derived cardiomyocytes generated from CPVT1 and CPVT2 patients carrying ryanodine or calsequestrin mutations. Journal of Cellular and Molecular Medicine. 2015;**19**(8):2006-2018

[27] Campuzano O, Sarquella-Brugada G, Brugada R, Brugada J. Genetics of channelopathies associated with sudden

cardiac death. Global Cardiology Science & Practice [Internet]. 2015;**2015**(3):39. Available from: http://www.qscience.com/doi/10.5339/gcsp.2015.39

[28] Venetucci L, Denegri M, Napolitano C, Priori SG. Inherited calcium channelopathies in the pathophysiology of arrhythmias. Nature Reviews. Cardiology. 2012;**9**:561-575

[29] Pérez-Riera AR, Barbosa-Barros R, de Rezende Barbosa MPC, Daminello-Raimundo R, de Lucca AA, de Abreu LC. Catecholaminergic polymorphic ventricular tachycardia, an update. Annals of Noninvasive Electrocardiology. 2018;**23**:e12512

[30] Pölönen RP, Penttinen K, Swan H, Aalto-Setälä K. Antiarrhythmic effects of carvedilol and flecainide in cardiomyocytes derived from catecholaminergic polymorphic ventricular tachycardia patients. Stem Cells International [Internet]. 2018;**2018**:1-11. Available from: https://www.hindawi.com/journals/sci/2018/9109503/

[31] Penttinen K, Swan H, Vanninen S, Paavola J, Lahtinen AM, Kontula K, et al. Antiarrhythmic effects of dantrolene in patients with catecholaminergic polymorphic ventricular tachycardia and replication of the responses using iPSC models. PLoS One. 2015;**10**(5):e0134746

[32] Zhang XH, Haviland S, Wei H, Šarić T, Fatima A, Hescheler J, et al. $Ca^{2+}$ signaling in human induced pluripotent stem cell-derived cardiomyocytes (iPS-CM) from normal and catecholaminergic polymorphic ventricular tachycardia (CPVT)-afflicted subjects. Cell Calcium. 2013;**54**(2):57-70

[33] Wei H, Zhang XH, Clift C, Yamaguchi N, Morad M. CRISPR/Cas9 Gene editing of RyR2 in human stem cell-derived cardiomyocytes provides a novel approach in investigating dysfunctional $Ca^{2+}$ signaling. Cell Calcium. 2018;**73**:104-111

[34] Van Der Werf C, Kannankeril PJ, Sacher F, Krahn AD, Viskin S, Leenhardt A, et al. Flecainide therapy reduces exercise-induced ventricular arrhythmias in patients with catecholaminergic polymorphic ventricular tachycardia. Journal of the American College of Cardiology. 2011;**57**(22):2244-2254

[35] Preininger MK, Jha R, Maxwell JT, Wu Q, Singh M, Wang B, et al. A human pluripotent stem cell model of catecholaminergic polymorphic ventricular tachycardia recapitulates patient-specific drug responses. Disease Models & Mechanisms [Internet]. 2016;**9**(9):927-939 Available from: http://dmm.biologists.org/lookup/doi/10.1242/dmm.026823

[36] Di Barletta MR, Viatchenko-Karpinski S, Nori A, Memmi M, Terentyev D, Turcato F, et al. Clinical phenotype and functional characterization of CASQ2 mutations associated with catecholaminergic polymorphic ventricular tachycardia. Circulation. 2006;**114**(10):1012-1019

[37] Lodola F, Morone D, Denegri M, Bongianino R, Nakahama H, Rutigliano L, et al. Adeno-associated virus-mediated CASQ2 delivery rescues phenotypic alterations in a patient-specific model of recessive catecholaminergic polymorphic ventricular tachycardia. Cell Death & Disease. 2016;**7**(10)

[38] Giudicessi JR, Ackerman MJ. Potassium-channel mutations and cardiac arrhythmias—Diagnosis and therapy. Nature Reviews. Cardiology. 2012;**9**:319-332

[39] Morita H, Wu J, Zipes DP. The QT syndromes: Long and short. The Lancet. 2008;**372**:750-763

[40] Ma D, Wei H, Lu J, Huang D, Liu Z, Loh LJ, et al. Characterization of a novel KCNQ1 mutation for type 1 long QT syndrome and assessment of the therapeutic potential of a novel IKs activator using patient-specific induced pluripotent stem cell-derived cardiomyocytes. Stem Cell Research & Therapy. 2015;**6**(1):39

[41] Sogo T, Morikawa K, Kurata Y, Li P, Ichinose T, Yuasa S, et al. Electrophysiological properties of iPS cell-derived cardiomyocytes from a patient with long QT syndrome type 1 harboring the novel mutation M437V of KCNQ1. Regenerative Therapy. 2016;**4**:9-17

[42] Moretti A, Bellin M, Welling A, Jung CB, Lam JT, Bott-Flügel L, et al. Patient-specific induced pluripotent stem-cell models for long-QT syndrome. New England Journal of Medicine [Internet]. 2010;**363**(15):1397-1409. Available from: http://www.nejm.org/doi/abs/10.1056/NEJMoa0908679

[43] Ahn J, Kim HJ, Choi J-I, Lee KN, Shim J, Ahn HS, et al. Effectiveness of beta-blockers depending on the genotype of congenital long-QT syndrome: A meta-analysis. PLoS One. 2017;**12**(10):e0185680

[44] Kubota T, Shimizu W, Kamakura S, Horie M. Hypokalemia-induced long QT syndrome with an underlying novel missense mutation in S4-S5 linker of KCNQ1. Journal of Cardiovascular Electrophysiology. 2000;**11**(9):1048-1054

[45] Kuusela J, Larsson K, Shah D, Prajapati C, Aalto-Setälä K. Low extracellular potassium prolongs repolarization and evokes early afterdepolarization in human induced pluripotent stem cell-derived cardiomyocytes. Biology Open [Internet]. 2017;**6**(6):777-784. Available from: http://bio.biologists.org/lookup/doi/10.1242/bio.024216

[46] Kiviaho AL, Ahola A, Larsson K, Penttinen K, Swan H, Pekkanen-Mattila M, et al. Distinct electrophysiological and mechanical beating phenotypes of long QT syndrome type 1-specific cardiomyocytes carrying different mutations. IJC Heart and Vasculature. 2015;**8**:19-31

[47] Ahola A, Kiviaho AL, Larsson K, Honkanen M, Aalto-Setälä K, Hyttinen J. Video image-based analysis of single human induced pluripotent stem cell derived cardiomyocyte beating dynamics using digital image correlation. Biomedical Engineering Online. 2014;**13**(1):39

[48] Matsa E, Rajamohan D, Dick E, Young L, Mellor I, Staniforth A, et al. Drug evaluation in cardiomyocytes derived from human induced pluripotent stem cells carrying a long QT syndrome type 2 mutation. European Heart Journal. 2011;**32**(8):952-962

[49] Itzhaki I, Maizels L, Huber I, Zwi-Dantsis L, Caspi O, Winterstern A, et al. Modelling the long QT syndrome with induced pluripotent stem cells. Nature. 2011;**471**(7337):225-230

[50] Lahti AL, Kujala VJ, Chapman H, Koivisto A-P, Pekkanen-Mattila M, Kerkelä E, et al. Model for long QT syndrome type 2 using human iPS cells demonstrates arrhythmogenic characteristics in cell culture. Disease Models & Mechanisms [Internet]. 2012;**5**(2):220-230. Available from: http://www.pubmedcentral.nih.gov/articlerender.fcgi?artid=3291643&tool=pmcentrez&rendertype=abstract

[51] Garg P, Oikonomopoulos A, Chen H, Li Y, Lam CK, Sallam K, et al. Genome editing of induced pluripotent stem cells to decipher cardiac channelopathy variant. Journal of the American College of Cardiology. 2018;**72**(1):62-75

[52] Mehta A, Sequiera GL, Ramachandra CJA, Sudibyo Y, Chung Y, Sheng J, et al. Re-trafficking of hERG reverses long QT syndrome 2 phenotype in human iPS-derived cardiomyocytes. Cardiovascular Research. 2014;**102**(3):497-506

[53] Sala L, Yu Z, Ward-Van Oostwaard D, Pd Van Veldhoven J, Moretti A, Laugwitz K-L, et al. A new hERG allosteric modulator rescues genetic and drug-induced long-QT syndrome phenotypes in cardiomyocytes from isogenic pairs of patient induced pluripotent stem cells. EMBO Molecular Medicine. 2016;**8**:1065-1081

[54] Matsa E, Dixon JE, Medway C, Georgiou O, Patel MJ, Morgan K, et al. Allele-specific RNA interference rescues the long-QT syndrome phenotype in human-induced pluripotency stem cell cardiomyocytes. European Heart Journal. 2014;**35**(16):1078-1087

[55] Bellin M, Casini S, Davis RP, D'Aniello C, Haas J, Ward-Van Oostwaard D, et al. Isogenic human pluripotent stem cell pairs reveal the role of a KCNH2 mutation in long-QT syndrome. The EMBO Journal. 2013;**32**(24):3161-3175

[56] Wang Q, Shen J, Splawski I, Atkinson D, Li Z, Robinson JL, et al. SCN5A mutations associated with an inherited cardiac arrhythmia, long QT syndrome. Cell. 1995;**80**(5):805-811

[57] Schwartz PJ, Priori SG, Spazzolini C, Moss AJ, Michael Vincent G, Napolitano C, et al. Genotype-phenotype correlation in the long-QT syndrome: Gene-specific triggers for life-threatening arrhythmias. Circulation. 2001;**103**(1):89-95

[58] Ma D, Wei H, Zhao Y, Lu J, Li G, Sahib NBE, et al. Modeling type 3 long QT syndrome with cardiomyocytes derived from patient-specific induced pluripotent stem cells. International Journal of Cardiology. 2013;**168**(6):5277-5286

[59] Malan D, Zhang M, Stallmeyer B, Müller J, Fleischmann BK, Schulze-Bahr E, et al. Human iPS cell model of type 3 long QT syndrome recapitulates drug-based phenotype correction. Basic Research in Cardiology. 2016;**111**(2):1-11

[60] Terrenoire C, Wang K, Chan Tung KW, Chung WK, Pass RH, Lu JT, et al. Induced pluripotent stem cells used to reveal drug actions in a long QT syndrome family with complex genetics. The Journal of General Physiology [Internet]. 2013;**141**(1):61-72. Available from: http://www.jgp.org/lookup/doi/10.1085/jgp.201210899

[61] Liang P, Sallam K, Wu H, Li Y, Itzhaki I, Garg P, et al. Patient-specific and genome-edited induced pluripotent stem cell–derived cardiomyocytes elucidate single-cell phenotype of Brugada syndrome. Journal of the American College of Cardiology. 2016;**68**(19):2086-2096

[62] Veerman CC, Mengarelli I, Guan K, Stauske M, Barc J, Tan HL, et al. HiPSC-derived cardiomyocytes from Brugada syndrome patients without identified mutations do not exhibit clear cellular electrophysiological abnormalities. Scientific Reports. 2016;**6**:30967

[63] Kosmidis G, Veerman CC, Casini S, Verkerk AO, Van De Pas S, Bellin M, et al. Readthrough-promoting drugs gentamicin and PTC124 Fail to Rescue Na v 1.5 function of human-induced pluripotent stem cell-derived cardiomyocytes carrying nonsense mutations in the sodium channel gene SCN5A. Circulation. Arrhythmia and Electrophysiology. 2016;**9**(11):e004227

[64] Zhang L, Benson DW, Tristani-Firouzi M, Ptacek LJ, Tawil R, Schwartz PJ, et al. Electrocardiographic features in Andersen-Tawil syndrome patients with KCNJ2 mutations: Characteristic

T-U-wave patterns predict the KCNJ2 genotype. Circulation. 2005;**111**(21): 2720-2726

[65] Kuroda Y, Yuasa S, Watanabe Y, Ito S, Egashira T, Seki T, et al. Flecainide ameliorates arrhythmogenicity through NCX flux in Andersen-Tawil syndrome-iPS cell-derived cardiomyocytes. Biochemistry and Biophysics Reports. 2017;**9**:245-256

[66] Splawski I, Timothy KW, Sharpe LM, Decher N, Kumar P, Bloise R, et al. CaV1.2 calcium channel dysfunction causes a multisystem disorder including arrhythmia and autism. Cell. 2004;**119**(1):19-31

[67] Yazawa M, Hsueh B, Jia X, Pasca AM, Bernstein JA, Hallmayer J, et al. Using iPS cells to investigate cardiac phenotypes in patients with Timothy syndrome. Nature [Internet]. 2011;**471**(7337):230-234. Available from: http://www.ncbi.nlm.nih.gov/pmc/articles/PMC3077925/

[68] Pérez-Riera AR, Paixão-Almeida A, Barbosa-Barros R, Yanowitz FG, Baranchuk A, Dubner S, et al. Congenital short QT syndrome: Landmarks of the newest arrhythmogenic cardiac channelopathy. Cardiology Journal. 2013;**20**:464-471

[69] Guerrier K, Kwiatkowski D, Czosek RJ, Spar DS, Anderson JB, Knilans TK. Short QT interval prevalence and clinical outcomes in a pediatric population. Circulation. Arrhythmia and Electrophysiology. 2015;**8**(6):1460-1464

[70] El-Battrawy I, Lan H, Cyganek L, Zhao Z, Li X, Buljubasic F, et al. Modeling short QT syndrome using human-induced pluripotent stem cell-derived cardiomyocytes. Journal of the American Heart Association. 2018;**7**(7):e007394

[71] Sisakian H. Cardiomyopathies: Evolution of pathogenesis concepts and potential for new therapies. World Journal of Cardiology [Internet]. 2014;**6**(6):478. Available from: http://www.wjgnet.com/1949-8462/full/v6/i6/478.htm

[72] Van Tintelen JP, Pieper PG, Van Spaendonck-Zwarts KY, Van Den Berg MP. Pregnancy, cardiomyopathies, and genetics. Cardiovascular Research. 2014;**101**:571-578

[73] Maron BJ. Hypertrophic cardiomyopathy. Circulation. 2002;**106**(19):2419-2421

[74] Pisano A, Cerbelli B, Perli E, Pelullo M, Bargelli V, Preziuso C, et al. Impaired mitochondrial biogenesis is a common feature to myocardial hypertrophy and end-stage ischemic heart failure. Cardiovascular Pathology. 2016;**25**(2):103-112

[75] Lan F, Lee AS, Liang P, Sanchez-Freire V, Nguyen PK, Wang L, et al. Abnormal calcium handling properties underlie familial hypertrophic cardiomyopathy pathology in patient-specific induced pluripotent stem cells. Cell Stem Cell. 2013;**12**(1):101-113

[76] Han L, Li Y, Tchao J, Kaplan AD, Lin B, Li Y, et al. Study familial hypertrophic cardiomyopathy using patient-specific induced pluripotent stem cells. Cardiovascular Research. 2014;**104**(2):258-269

[77] Tanaka A, Yuasa S, Mearini G, Egashira T, Seki T, Kodaira M, et al. Endothelin-1 induces myofibrillar disarray and contractile vector variability in hypertrophic cardiomyopathy-induced pluripotent stem cell-derived cardiomyocytes. Journal of the American Heart Association. 2014;**3**(6):e001263

[78] Prajapati C, Ojala M, Aalto-Setälä K. Divergent effect of adrenaline in human induced pluripotent stem cell derived cardiomyocytes obtained from

hypertrophic cardiomyopathy. Disease Models & Mechanisms [Internet]. 2018;**11**:dmm.032896. Available from: http://www.ncbi.nlm.nih.gov/pubmed/29361520

[79] Marston S, Copeland O, Jacques A, Livesey K, Tsang V, McKenna WJ, et al. Evidence from human myectomy samples that MYBPC3 mutations cause hypertrophic cardiomyopathy through haploinsufficiency. Circulation Research. 2009;**105**(3):219-222

[80] Prondzynski M, Krämer E, Laufer SD, Shibamiya A, Pless O, Flenner F, et al. Evaluation of MYBPC3 trans-splicing and gene replacement as therapeutic options in human iPSC-derived cardiomyocytes. Molecular Therapy—Nucleic Acids. 2017;7:475-486

[81] Song W, Dyer E, Stuckey DJ, Copeland O, Leung MC, Bayliss C, et al. Molecular mechanism of the E99K mutation in cardiac actin (ACTC gene) that causes apical hypertrophy in man and mouse. The Journal of Biological Chemistry. 2011;**286**(31):27582-27593

[82] Smith JGW, Owen T, Bhagwan JR, Mosqueira D, Scott E, Mannhardt I, et al. Isogenic pairs of hiPSC-CMs with hypertrophic cardiomyopathy/LVNC-associated ACTC1 E99K mutation unveil differential functional deficits. Stem Cell Reports. 2018;**11**(5):1226-1243

[83] Knollmann BC, Kirchhof P, Sirenko SG, Degen H, Greene AE, Schober T, et al. Familial hypertrophic cardiomyopathy-linked mutant troponin T causes stress-induced ventricular tachycardia and $Ca^{2+}$-dependent action potential remodeling. Circulation Research. 2003;**92**(4):428-436

[84] Wang L, Kim K, Parikh S, Cadar AG, Bersell KR, He H, et al. Hypertrophic cardiomyopathy-linked mutation in troponin T causes myofibrillar disarray and pro-arrhythmic action potential changes in human iPSC cardiomyocytes. Journal of Molecular and Cellular Cardiology. 2018;**114**:320-327

[85] Hedman A, Hartikainen J, Vanninen E, Laitinen T, Jääskeläinen P, Laakso M, et al. Inducibility of life-threatening ventricular arrhythmias is related to maximum left ventricular thickness and clinical markers of sudden cardiac death in patients with hypertrophic cardiomyopathy attributable to the Asp175Asn mutation in the α-tropomyosin. Journal of Molecular and Cellular Cardiology. 2004;**36**(1):91-99

[86] Li S, Pan H, Tan C, Sun Y, Song Y, Zhang X, et al. Mitochondrial dysfunctions contribute to hypertrophic cardiomyopathy in patient iPSC-derived cardiomyocytes with MT-RNR2 mutation. Stem Cell Reports. 2018;**10**(3):808-821

[87] Hershberger RE, Siegfried JD. Update 2011: Clinical and genetic issues in familial dilated cardiomyopathy. Journal of the American College of Cardiology. 2011;**57**(16):1641-1649

[88] Beraldi R, Li X, Fernandez AM, Reyes S, Secreto F, Terzic A, et al. Rbm20-deficient cardiogenesis reveals early disruption of RNA processing and sarcomere remodeling establishing a developmental etiology for dilated cardiomyopathy. Human Molecular Genetics. 2014;**23**(14):3779-3791

[89] Streckfuss-Bömeke K, Tiburcy M, Fomin A, Luo X, Li W, Fischer C, et al. Severe DCM phenotype of patient harboring RBM20 mutation S635A can be modeled by patient-specific induced pluripotent stem cell-derived cardiomyocytes. Journal of Molecular and Cellular Cardiology. 2017;**113**:9-21

[90] Wyles SP, Li X, Hrstka SC, Reyes S, Oommen S, Beraldi R, et al. Modeling structural and functional deficiencies of

RBM20 familial dilated cardiomyopathy using human induced pluripotent stem cells. Human Molecular Genetics. 2016;**25**(2):254-265

[91] Guo W, Schafer S, Greaser ML, Radke MH, Liss M, Govindarajan T, et al. RBM20, a gene for hereditary cardiomyopathy, regulates titin splicing. Nature Medicine. 2012;**18**(5):766-773

[92] Hershberger RE, Pinto JR, Parks SB, Kushner JD, Li D, Ludwigsen S, et al. Clinical and functional characterization of TNNT2 mutations identified in patients with dilated cardiomyopathy. Circulation. Cardiovascular Genetics. 2009;**2**(4):306-313

[93] Sun N, Yazawa M, Liu J, Han L, Sanchez-Freire V, Abilez OJ, et al. Patient-specific induced pluripotent stem cells as a model for familial dilated cardiomyopathy. Science Translational Medicine. 2012;**4**(130):130ra47

[94] Song K, Dubé MP, Lim J, Hwang I, Lee I, Kim J-J. Lamin A/C mutations associated with familial and sporadic cases of dilated cardiomyopathy in Koreans. Experimental & Molecular Medicine [Internet]. 2007;**39**(1): 114-120. Available from: http://www.ncbi.nlm.nih.gov/pubmed/17334235

[95] Siu CW, Lee YK, Ho JCY, Lai WH, Chan YC, Ng KM, et al. Modeling of lamin A/C mutation premature cardiac aging using patient-specific induced pluripotent stem cells. Aging. 2012;**4**(11):803-822

[96] Tse HF, Ho JCY, Choi SW, Lee YK, Butler AW, Ng KM, et al. Patient-specific induced-pluripotent stem cells-derived cardiomyocytes recapitulate the pathogenic phenotypes of dilated cardiomyopathy due to a novel DES mutation identified by whole exome sequencing. Human Molecular Genetics. 2013;**22**(7):1395-1403

[97] Van Der Zwaag PA, Van Rijsingen IAW, Asimaki A, Jongbloed JDH, Van Veldhuisen DJ, Wiesfeld ACP, et al. Phospholamban R14del mutation in patients diagnosed with dilated cardiomyopathy or arrhythmogenic right ventricular cardiomyopathy: Evidence supporting the concept of arrhythmogenic cardiomyopathy. European Journal of Heart Failure. 2012;**14**(11):1199-1207

[98] Karakikes I, Stillitano F, Nonnenmacher M, Tzimas C, Sanoudou D, Termglinchan V, et al. Correction of human phospholamban R14del mutation associated with cardiomyopathy using targeted nucleases and combination therapy. Nature Communications. 2015;**6**:6955

[99] Stillitano F, Turnbull IC, Karakikes I, Nonnenmacher M, Backeris P, Hulot JS, et al. Genomic correction of familial cardiomyopathy in human engineered cardiac tissues. European Heart Journal. 2016;**37**(43):3282-3284

[100] Sommariva E, Stadiotti I, Perrucci GL, Tondo C, Pompilio G. Cell models of arrhythmogenic cardiomyopathy: Advances and opportunities. Disease Models & Mechanisms [Internet]. 2017;**10**(7):823-835. Available from: http://dmm.biologists.org/lookup/doi/10.1242/dmm.029363

[101] Asimaki A, Tandri H, Huang H, Halushka MK, Gautam S, Basso C, et al. A new diagnostic test for arrhythmogenic right ventricular cardiomyopathy. New England Journal of Medicine [Internet]. 2009;**360**(11):1075-1084. Available from: http://www.nejm.org/doi/abs/10.1056/NEJMoa0808138

[102] Ma D, Wei H, Lu J, Ho S, Zhang G, Sun X, et al. Generation of patient-specific induced pluripotent stem cell-derived cardiomyocytes as a cellular model of arrhythmogenic right ventricular cardiomyopathy. European Heart Journal. 2013;**34**(15):1122-1133

[103] Caspi O, Huber I, Gepstein A, Arbel G, Maizels L, Boulos M, et al. Modeling of arrhythmogenic right ventricular cardiomyopathy with human induced pluripotent stem cells. Circulation. Cardiovascular Genetics. 2013;**6**(6):557-568

[104] Kim C, Wong J, Wen J, Wang S, Wang C, Spiering S, et al. Studying arrhythmogenic right ventricular dysplasia with patient-specific iPSCs. Nature. 2013;**494**(7435):105-110

[105] Bauce B, Frigo G, Marcus FI, Basso C, Rampazzo A, Maddalena F, et al. Comparison of clinical features of arrhythmogenic right ventricular cardiomyopathy in men versus women. The American Journal of Cardiology. 2008;**102**(9):1252-1257

[106] Akdis D, Saguner AM, Shah K, Wei C, Medeiros-Domingo A, Von Eckardstein A, et al. Sex hormones affect outcome in arrhythmogenic right ventricular cardiomyopathy/dysplasia: From a stem cell derived cardiomyocyte-based model to clinical biomarkers of disease outcome. European Heart Journal. 2017;**38**(19):1498-1508

[107] Prajapati C, Pölönen R-P, Aalto-Setälä K. Simultaneous recordings of action potentials and calcium transients from human induced pluripotent stem cell derived cardiomyocytes. Biology Open [Internet]. 2018;7(7):bio035030. Available from: http://bio.biologists.org/content/early/2018/06/20/bio.035030.abstract

[108] Jung CB, Moretti A, Mederos y Schnitzler M, Iop L, Storch U, Bellin M, et al. Dantrolene rescues arrhythmogenic RYR2 defect in a patient-specific stem cell model of catecholaminergic polymorphic ventricular tachycardia. EMBO Molecular Medicine. 2012;**4**(3):180-191

[109] Tiburcy M, Hudson JE, Balfanz P, Schlick S, Meyer T, Liao MLC, et al. Defined engineered human myocardium with advanced maturation for applications in heart failure modeling and repair. Circulation. 2017;**135**(19):1832-1847

[110] Lemoine MD, Mannhardt I, Breckwoldt K, Prondzynski M, Flenner F, Ulmer B, et al. Human iPSC-derived cardiomyocytes cultured in 3D engineered heart tissue show physiological upstroke velocity and sodium current density. Scientific Reports. 2017;**7**(1)

[111] Correia C, Koshkin A, Duarte P, Hu D, Carido M, Sebastião MJ, et al. 3D aggregate culture improves metabolic maturation of human pluripotent stem cell derived cardiomyocytes. Biotechnology and Bioengineering [Internet]. 2017;**115**(3):360-644. Available from: http://doi.wiley.com/10.1002/bit.26504

[112] Shadrin IY, Allen BW, Qian Y, Jackman CP, Carlson AL, Juhas ME, et al. Cardiopatch platform enables maturation and scale-up of human pluripotent stem cell-derived engineered heart tissues. Nature Communications. 2017;**8**(1):1825

[113] Amin AS, Tan HL, Wilde AAM. Cardiac ion channels in health and disease. Heart Rhythm [Internet]. 2010;**7**(1):117-126. Available from: http://www.sciencedirect.com/science/article/pii/S1547527109008443

[114] Dobrev D, Nattel S. New antiarrhythmic drugs for treatment of atrial fibrillation. The Lancet. 2010;**375**:1212-1223

[115] Lee JH, Protze SI, Laksman Z, Backx PH, Keller GM. Human pluripotent stem cell-derived atrial and ventricular cardiomyocytes develop from distinct mesoderm populations. Cell Stem Cell. 2017;**21**(2):179-194.e4

[116] Choudhury M, Boyett MR, Morris GM. Biology of the sinus

node and its disease. Arrhythmia & Electrophysiology Review [Internet]. 2015;**4**(1):28. Available from: http://www.radcliffecardiology.com/articles/biology-sinus-node-and-its-disease

[117] Protze SI, Liu J, Nussinovitch U, Ohana L, Backx PH, Gepstein L, et al. Sinoatrial node cardiomyocytes derived from human pluripotent cells function as a biological pacemaker. Nature Biotechnology. 2017;**35**(1):56-68

[118] Shamis Y, Hewitt KJ, Bear SE, Addy AH, Qari H, Margvelashvilli M, et al. IPSC-derived fibroblasts demonstrate augmented production and assembly of extracellular matrix proteins. In Vitro Cellular & Developmental Biology—Animal. 2012;**48**(2):112-122

[119] Orlova VV, Van Den Hil FE, Petrus-Reurer S, Drabsch Y, Ten Dijke P, Mummery CL. Generation, expansion and functional analysis of endothelial cells and pericytes derived from human pluripotent stem cells. Nature Protocols. 2014;**9**(6):1514-1531

[120] Granata A, Serrano F, Bernard WG, McNamara M, Low L, Sastry P, et al. An iPSC-derived vascular model of Marfan syndrome identifies key mediators of smooth muscle cell death. Nature Genetics. 2017;**49**(1):97-109

[121] Musunuru K. Genome editing of human pluripotent stem cells to generate human cellular disease models. Disease Models & Mechanisms [Internet]. 2013;**6**(4):896-904. Available from: http://dmm.biologists.org/cgi/doi/10.1242/dmm.012054

Section 3

# Myocardial Metabolics

Chapter 6

# Obesity-Related Myocardiopathy

*Marco Antonio Lopez Hernandez*

## Abstract

Cardiovascular disease in populations with obesity is a major concern because of it is epidemic proportion. Obesity leads to the development of cardiomyopathy directly via inflammatory mediators and indirectly by obesity-induced hypertension, diabetes, and coronary artery diseases. Metabolic disturbances such as increased free fatty acid levels, insulin resistance, elevated levels of adipokines, myocardial remodeling, activation of the sympathetic nervous and renin-angiotensin-aldosterone systems, and small-vessel disease are the most important mechanisms in the development of obesity cardiomyopathy. The myocardial changes related with obesity are increasingly recognized, and they are independent of classic risk factors as hypertension, coronary artery disease, and obstructive sleep apnea. There is a wide range of evidence: the association between heart failure and obesity shown in epidemiologic studies; the confirmation of the association of adiposity with left ventricular dysfunction, independent of hypertension, coronary artery disease, and other heart diseases; and experimental evidence of functional and structural changes in the myocardium in response to increased adiposity support the existence of a cardiomyopathy related to obesity.

**Keywords:** heart failure, obesity, adipokines, myocardiopathy

## 1. Introduction

During the past half-century, the advances in the prevention, diagnosis, and management of cardiovascular disease (CVD) have been spectacular. The cardiovascular-related deaths have declined by about two-thirds in industrialized nations [1].

Heart failure is characterized by an increased rate of cell death, which has been attributed to a variety of conditions: oxidative stress; abnormal elevations in circulating neurohormones; toxins, such as alcohol or cancer chemotherapeutic drugs; excessive adrenergic activity; inflammation; and infiltrative processes. Apoptosis is a highly regulated type of cell death that normally increases with aging. It has been suggested that, over time, the resulting deletion of myocytes leads to heart failure [2, 3].

The metabolic demand is increased in obesity; this is due to different factors as increasing blood volume, greater adipose tissue and lean mass, and as such, increased preload to the heart. In addition, in obese patients there are vascular alterations impacting arterial stiffness, and resistance increases afterload to the heart. In adults with obesity, both eccentric and concentric hypertrophies have been noted and are impacted by the duration and the degree of the obesity [4, 5].



IntechOpen

## 2. Regional adiposity and cardiovascular risk

While the cardiovascular risk is linked to the adipose tissue quantity, recent data indicate that differences in fat tissue quality, which can be examined directly by noninvasive computed tomography radiodensity attenuation imaging or by immunohistochemistry, are closely linked to insulin resistance, cardiometabolic risk, and all-cause mortality, independent of total fat volume. These data demonstrate, independent of body mass index, that abnormalities at the adipose tissue level may be key factors that regulate systemic metabolism and drive cardiometabolic disease. These qualitative abnormalities in fat are a growing area of research interest that have been recently termed sick fat or adiposopathy and may in part explain the clinical observation of metabolically healthy obesity. The interindividual variability in adipose tissue "quality" may be related, in part, to differences in lifestyle, as physical activity has effects on adipose tissue physiology and cardiometabolic risk. While animal models of obesity tend to generate fairly uniform phenotypes, the degree of adipose tissue dysfunction in obese humans exhibits significant heterogeneity with lower degrees of adiposopathy being associated with more favorable systemic metabolic profiles and vascular function.

## 3. Adipokines, myokines, and cardiovascular disease

It is recognized that obesity contributes to cardiovascular and metabolic disorders through alterations in the levels of adipocyte-derived cytokines that are named adipokines.

The functions of adipose tissue are as energy storage and as secretory tissue producing a variety of bioactive substances, including leptin, tumor necrosis factor alpha (TNFα), plasminogen activator inhibitor type 1, and adiponectin [6–9]. These bioactive molecules are generally referred to as adipokines, and several are involved in the pathophysiology of various obesity-linked disorders.

## 4. Leptin

Leptin is an adipose tissue-specific-secreted hormone and is highly expressed by adipocytes; this adipokine is encoded by the ob gene, which was identified in genetically obese ob/ob mice through positional cloning. The circulating leptin levels increase in parallel to adipose tissue mass. Leptin exerts important metabolic actions by suppressing appetite and increasing energy expenditure. Many lines of evidence suggest that hyperleptinemia contributes to cardiovascular complications. Leptin has pro-inflammatory actions in many immune cell types including monocytes/macrophage, neutrophils, NK cells, and T cells [10–17].

## 5. Adiponectin

Adiponectin is abundantly present in human plasma at a range between 3 and 30 μg/mL. It is an adipokine whose mRNA is largely expressed in adipose tissue. Adiponectin multimerizes to form stable higher-order complexes and shares structural homology with the collectin family of proteins.

Lower plasma levels of adiponectin are implicated in the pathogenesis of obesity-related diseases [18–21]. Conversely, plasma adiponectin concentrations increase following weight loss [22, 23]. In patients with diabetes mellitus, the levels of adiponectin are lower than patients without diabetes matched for age and weight [14]. An inverse correlation has been demonstrated between circulating levels of adiponectin and those as C-reactive protein and interleukin 6 [24–27].

Adiponectin appears to protect against the development of various vascular diseases. In murine experiments, it has been demonstrated that adiponectin has an anti-atherogenic function. In apolipoprotein E-deficient mice, the administration of an adenovirus-expressing adiponectin reduces atherosclerotic lesion size [28]. In apolipoprotein E-deficient mice, the adiponectin deficit leads to an increase in vascular lesion area [29]. Adiponectin knockout mice also develop increased neointimal thickness and display increased vascular smooth muscle cell proliferation following acute arterial injury, whereas overexpression of adiponectin inhibits neointimal lesion formation in wild-type mice [30].

Experimental studies have found that adiponectin exerts beneficial actions on the heart under pathological conditions. Adiponectin-deficient mice develop severe cardiac hypertrophy, and there is increased mortality in response to pressure overload because of transverse aortic constriction [31, 32].

## 6. Interleukin 6

Interleukin 6 (IL-6) is known to be secreted by several tissues; it is a pleiotropic cytokine with complex roles in metabolic and cardiovascular disease. IL-6 also can act in a local fashion. However, adipose tissue is a major source of this protein, capable of producing high levels of this protein in the blood. It has been estimated that as much as one-third of total circulating IL-6 originates from adipose tissue. Therefore, IL-6 can be considered an adipokine with endocrine actions.

IL-6-induced cell signaling is typically classified as either classic or trans-signaling, and it can lead to different cell responses. In the classic signaling way, the target cells are stimulated by IL-6 stimulates via a membrane-bound IL-6 receptor (IL6R), which upon ligand binding forms a complex with the signaling receptor protein gp130. Essentially all cells exhibit gp130 on the cell surface, whereas few cell types express membrane-bound IL6R. While the cells that only express gp130 are not responsive to IL-6 alone, they can be stimulated, via trans-signaling, by a complex of IL-6 bound to a naturally occurring soluble form of IL6R (sIL6R), markedly expanding the spectrum of IL-6 actions and target cells.

## 7. Resistin

Resistin is highly expressed by mature adipocytes in rodents. This adipokine is a secreted protein that was initially suggested to be a major link between insulin resistance and obesity. Circulating resistin levels are increased in diabetic and obese mice, and the important role of resistin in metabolic dysfunction associated with obesity through pleiotropic effects on insulin sensitivity and glucose metabolism has been suggested in several loss- and gain-of-function studies in mice .

## 8. Myokines

Myokines have been defined as cytokines and proteins produced and released by myocytes under the action of contractile activity. They exert an autocrine, paracrine, or endocrine effect. Their receptors were found in the muscle, fat, liver, pancreas, bone tissue, heart, brain, and immune cells [33, 34].

Although the endocrine function of adipose tissue has long been recognized, most of the factors produced are pro-inflammatory and harmful in the setting of obesity-induced metabolic disorders and cardiovascular disease. In this regard, adiponectin is relatively unique as an adipokine because it is expressed at highest levels in lean, healthy individuals.

Candidate cDNAs that encode secreted proteins and are differentially regulated in the muscle of the MyoMouse model are then used to construct adenoviral vectors for further testing in animal models of disease. One such factor, follistatin-like 1 (Fstl1), was identified in this type of screen and shown to have cardiovascular-protective properties. Fstl1, also referred to as TSC36, is an extracellular glycoprotein that has been grouped into the follistatin family of proteins [35].

The main myokines studied to date are myostatin, decorin, irisin, myonectin, interleukin-6 (IL-6), interleukin-8 (IL-8), interleukin-15 (IL-15), follistatin, fibroblast growth factor 21 (FGF21), bone morphogenetic protein (BMP), and brain-derived neurotrophic factor (BDNF). Other possible factors have been detected in the skeletal muscle, but their functions, as well as their presence in the circulation, are largely unknown: musclin and nonneuronal acetylcholine.

## 9. Myostatin

Also called growth differentiation factor 8 (GDF-8), it is a member of the transforming growth factor-β (TGF-β) family, expressed in developing and adult muscular tissue. It is one of the first described myokines.

Its main function is the negative regulation of the muscle mass, which means high level of myostatin and less muscle mass. It plays a role in stopping myoblast proliferation and suppressing satellite cell activation, inducing muscle atrophy. In addition, it influences the differentiation of muscle fibers by types (fast and slow) and the arrangement of muscle glucose as well as the muscle-adipose tissue cross-talking [36–40].

## 10. Irisin

Discovered in 2012 as a transmembrane protein, FNDC5 has a cleaved soluble form, irisin, that it is released into circulation during the proteolytic process after acute exercising of skeletal muscles. It increases the energetic and oxidative metabolism of the muscle by activating genes related to these processes. It has a high level during myogenesis and induces glucose uptake improving glucose homeostasis, inhibiting lipid accumulation, and reducing body weight [41, 42]. Irisin has been studied especially in relation to obesity but also with myopathies such as muscular dystrophy. In these latter studies, injection of irisin induced muscle hypertrophy, improving muscle strength and reducing necrosis and development of connective tissue in a murine model [42].

## 11. Myonectin

Myonectin is a protein belonging to the C1q/TNF-related protein (CTRP) family, and it is found mainly in the muscle, less in circulation, being especially related to nutritional metabolism. Thus, the expression of myonectin is stimulated by exercise and nutrients and is supposed to induce nutrient uptake and storage in other tissues, such as adipose tissue, causing a flux of glucose or fatty acids [42, 43].

## 12. Mechanism of myocardiopathy in obesity

Insulin resistance, adiposity, and adipokines have been implicated in the development of abnormal myocardial mechanics in adults with obesity and type 2 diabetes. Adiposopathy in obese individuals is ultimately the consequence of a dysfunctional remodeling of the adipose tissue. Therefore, for understanding how obesity contributes to cardiovascular disease, it is primordial to know how both quantitative and qualitative effects of this adipose tissue remodeling contribute to that.

## 13. Adipose tissue expansion

In response to an excessive caloric intake, the mechanisms by which adipose depots expand represent an important determinant of the risk of cardiovascular disease and metabolic dysfunction. This expansion is mediated by two ways: an enlargement of adipocyte size (hypertrophy) and/or an increase in adipocyte numbers (hyperplasia).

Adipocyte hypertrophy typically leads to lipid-laden, dysfunctional adipocytes that undergo cell death and contribute to adipose tissue inflammation, dysfunction, and associated pathologies; in contrast it has been classically accepted that hyperplasia allows a "healthy" expansion of the adipose tissue, since it is mediated by the formation of functional adipocytes from progenitor cells (adipogenesis).

## 14. Immune cell infiltration

In most cases chronic excessive caloric intake eventually leads to adipocyte dysfunction, regardless of the mechanisms of adipose tissue expansion, and this is paralleled by qualitative and quantitative changes in the composition of adipose tissue at cellular level. Immune cells are of great relevance in this regard. Low-grade chronic inflammation is a major hallmark of adipose tissue in obesity, and it is now known that almost every immune cell type can be found in the adipose tissue. Total numbers of B cells, T cells, neutrophils, macrophages, and mast cells are increased in visceral adipose tissue of obese individuals. In contrast, the number of eosinophils and specific subsets of T cells—T-helper type 2 (Th2) cells and regulatory T (Treg) cells—are decreased or remained static in the adipose tissue of obese individuals [36].

Macrophages are the most abundant immune cell in the adipose tissue of obese individuals, and their recruitment and proliferation upon high-calorie feeding is generally associated with adipose tissue inflammation and insulin resistance [44–47].

## 15. Impaired vascular structure and function

Several studies in humans and animal models have shown that obesity induces capillary rarefaction in adipose tissue, and this has been associated with metabolic dysfunction. It is widely a reduced adipose tissue; capillarization is present in obesity, and this reduced blood supply may limit nutrient delivery and contribute to adipocyte dysfunction and insulin resistance.

Evidence of a causal role of adipose tissue vascularization in obesity-associated metabolic dysfunction have been shown in recent studies with genetically engineered mice. Experiments demonstrated that an increased VEGF-mediated angiogenesis in adipose tissue can attenuate some of the metabolic effects of diet-induced obesity, such as insulin resistance and hepatic steatosis in mice overexpressing vascular endothelial growth factor A (VEGF-A) in adipocytes. Conversely, adipocyte-restricted deletion of VEGF-A results in diminished adipose tissue vascularization, which leads to increased adipose tissue inflammation and systemic metabolic dysfunction further supporting the noxious effects of reduced adipose tissue vascularity in obesity [48–51].

## 16. Adipose tissue fibrosis

Within the adipose tissue of lean organisms, adipocytes are surrounded by extracellular matrix that provides mechanical support and participates in cell signaling. There is a general increase in the synthesis of several extracellular matrix components with the development of obesity, in particular collagen VI, which leads to adipose tissue fibrosis and is associated with impaired metabolic function in mice. Adipose tissue fibrosis is increased in both subcutaneous and visceral depots in obesity. Obesity-induced adipose tissue fibrosis is due, at least in part, to hypoxia-induced upregulation of hypoxia-inducible factor 1α (HIF1α). Interestingly, HIF1α activation does not contribute to an angiogenic response in this context, but instead promotes adipose tissue fibrosis [52].

## 17. Conclusions

An increasing evidence supports the evolving concept that quality, quantity, and location of adipose tissue are critical factors in shaping cardiometabolic phenotypes in obese individuals. The specific pathogenic mechanisms and their relative contributions remain incompletely understood. Adipose tissue communicates with remote organs, including the heart and vasculature, through the release of various adipokines. While some adipokines have been highly studied and have shown to be causally linked to various disease processes, new adipokine candidates continue to be discovered and elucidated. In murine models and many human individuals, obesity leads to adipose tissue dysfunction; this dysfunction is termed adiposopathy, particularly in visceral fat depots, which is mediated by dysfunctional tissue remodeling that involves adipocyte hypertrophy, increased fibrosis exacerbated inflammation, and impaired vascular function and structure. This ultimately creates a chronic, low-grade systemic inflammatory reaction mediated by an imbalance in adipokine levels which contributes to the initiation and progression of metabolic and cardiovascular complications. As our understanding of adipokines and obesity-induced adiposopathy increases, the major challenge will reside in translating this information into new prognostic and therapeutic approaches to limit cardiovascular risk in obese individuals. Considering that a third of the world's population is currently overweight or obese and this proportion is expected to increase in the coming decades, studies of adipokine biology should provide a better understanding of the pathogenesis of cardiovascular disease.

## Author details

Marco Antonio Lopez Hernandez
Internal Medicine Division, Ecatepec General Hospital, Autonomous University of Mexico's State, State of Mexico, Mexico

*Address all correspondence to: niklaus2003@yahoo.com.mx

## References

[1] Nabel EG, Braunwald E. A tale of coronary artery disease and myocardial infarction. The New England Journal of Medicine. 2012;**366**(10):970

[2] Konstantinidis K, Whelan RS, Kitsis RN. Mechanisms of cell death in heart disease. Arteriosclerosis, Thrombosis, and Vascular Biology. 2012;**32**:1552-1562

[3] Olivetti G, Abbi R, Quaini F, et al. Apoptosis in the failing human heart. The New England Journal of Medicine. 1997;**336**:1131-1141

[4] Alpert MA. Obesity cardiomyopathy: Pathophysiology and evolution of the clinical syndrome. The American Journal of the Medical Sciences. 2001;**321**:225-236

[5] Vasan RS. Cardiac function and obesity. Heart. 2003;**89**:1127-1129

[6] Zhang Y, Proenca R, Maffei M, Barone M, Leopold L, Friedman JM. Positional cloning of the mouse obese gene and its human homologue. Nature. 1994;**372**:425-432

[7] Hotamisligil GS, Shargill NS, Spiegelman BM. Adipose expression of tumor necrosis factor-alpha: Direct role in obesity-linked insulin resistance. Science. 1993;**259**:87-91

[8] Shimomura I, Funahashi T, Takahashi M, Maeda K, Kotani K, Nakamura T, et al. Enhanced expression of PAI-1 in visceral fat: Possible contributor to vascular disease in obesity. Nature Medicine. 1996;**2**:800-803

[9] Maeda K, Okubo K, Shimomura I, Funahashi T, Matsuzawa Y, Matsubara K. cDNA cloning and expression of a novel adipose specific collagen-like factor, apM1 (AdiPose Most abundant gene transcript 1). Biochemical and Biophysical Research Communications. 1996;**221**:286-289

[10] Santos-Alvarez J, Goberna R, Sanchez-Margalet V. Human leptin stimulates proliferation and activation of human circulating monocytes. Cellular Immunology. 1999;**194**:6-11

[11] Surmi BK, Atkinson RD, Gruen ML, Coenen KR, Hasty AH. The role of macrophage leptin receptor in aortic root lesion formation. American Journal of Physiology. Endocrinology and Metabolism. 2008;**294**:E488-E495

[12] Kiguchi N, Maeda T, Kobayashi Y, Fukazawa Y, Kishioka S. Leptin enhances CC-chemokine ligand expression in cultured murine macrophage. Biochemical and Biophysical Research Communications. 2009;**384**:311-315

[13] Gainsford T, Willson TA, Metcalf D, Handman E, McFarlane C, Ng A, et al. Leptin can induce proliferation, differentiation, and functional activation of hemopoietic cells. Proceedings of the National Academy of Sciences of the United States of America. 1996;**93**:14564-14568

[14] Caldefie-Chezet F, Poulin A, Vasson MP. Leptin regulates functional capacities of polymorphonuclear neutrophils. Free Radical Research. 2003;**37**:809-814

[15] Tian Z, Sun R, Wei H, Gao B. Impaired natural killer (NK) cell activity in leptin receptor deficient mice: Leptin as a critical regulator in NK cell development and activation. Biochemical and Biophysical Research Communications. 2002;**298**:297-302

[16] Lord GM, Matarese G, Howard JK, Baker RJ, Bloom SR, Lechler RI. Leptin modulates the T-cell immune

response and reverses starvation-induced immunosuppression. Nature. 1998;**394**:897-901

[17] De Rosa V, Procaccini C, Cali G, Pirozzi G, Fontana S, Zappacosta S, et al. A key role of leptin in the control of regulatory T cell proliferation. Immunity. 2007;**26**:241-255

[18] Arita Y, Kihara S, Ouchi N, Takahashi M, Maeda K, Miyagawa J, et al. Paradoxical decrease of an adipose-specific protein, adiponectin, in obesity. Biochemical and Biophysical Research Communications. 1999;**257**:79-83

[19] Shapiro L, Scherer PE. The crystal structure of a complement-1q family protein suggests an evolutionary link to tumor necrosis factor. Current Biology. 1998;**8**:335-338

[20] Cnop M, Havel PJ, Utzschneider KM, Carr DB, Sinha MK, Boyko EJ, et al. Relationship of adiponectin to body fat distribution, insulin sensitivity and plasma lipoproteins: Evidence for independent roles of age and sex. Diabetologia. 2003;**46**:459-469

[21] Weyer C, Funahashi T, Tanaka S, Hotta K, Matsuzawa Y, Pratley RE, et al. Hypoadiponectinemia in obesity and type 2 diabetes: Close association with insulin resistance and hyperinsulinemia. The Journal of Clinical Endocrinology and Metabolism. 2001;**86**:1930-1935

[22] Hotta K, Funahashi T, Arita Y, Takahashi M, Matsuda M, Okamoto Y, et al. Plasma concentrations of a novel, adipose-specific protein, adiponectin, in type 2 diabetic patients. Arteriosclerosis, Thrombosis, and Vascular Biology. 2000;**20**:1595-1599

[23] Yang WS, Lee WJ, Funahashi T, Tanaka S, Matsuzawa Y, Chao CL, et al. Weight reduction increases plasma levels of an adipose-derived anti-inflammatory protein, adiponectin. The Journal of Clinical Endocrinology and Metabolism. 2001;**86**:3815-3819

[24] Ouchi N, Kihara S, Funahashi T, Nakamura T, Nishida M, Kumada M, et al. Reciprocal association of C-reactive protein with adiponectin in blood stream and adipose tissue. Circulation. 2003;**107**:671-674

[25] Engeli S, Feldpausch M, Gorzelniak K, Hartwig F, Heintze U, Janke J, et al. Association between adiponectin and mediators of inflammation in obese women. Diabetes. 2003;**52**:942-947

[26] Krakoff J, Funahashi T, Stehouwer CD, Schalkwijk CG, Tanaka S, Matsuzawa Y, et al. Inflammatory markers, adiponectin, and risk of type 2 diabetes in the Pima Indian. Diabetes Care. 2003;**26**:1745-1751

[27] Esposito K, Pontillo A, Di Palo C, Giugliano G, Masella M, Marfella R, et al. Effect of weight loss and lifestyle changes on vascular inflammatory markers in obese women: A randomized trial. JAMA. 2003;**289**:1799-1804

[28] Okamoto Y, Kihara S, Ouchi N, Nishida M, Arita Y, Kumada M, et al. Adiponectin reduces atherosclerosis in apolipoprotein E-deficient mice. Circulation. 2002;**106**:2767-2770

[29] Okamoto Y, Folco EJ, Minami M, Wara AK, Feinberg MW, Sukhova GK, et al. Adiponectin inhibits the production of CXC receptor 3 chemokine ligands in macrophages and reduces T-lymphocyte recruitment in atherogenesis. Circulation Research. 2008;**102**:218-225

[30] Matsuda M, Shimomura I, Sata M, Arita Y, Nishida M, Maeda N, et al. Role of adiponectin in preventing vascular stenosis: The missing link of adipo-vascular axis. The Journal of Biological Chemistry. 2002;**277**:37487-37491

[31] Shibata R, Ouchi N, Ito M, Kihara S, Shiojima I, Pimentel DR, et al. Adiponectin-mediated modulation of hypertrophic signals in the heart. Nature Medicine. 2004;**10**:1384-1389

[32] Liao Y, Takashima S, Maeda N, Ouchi N, Komamura K, Shimomura I, et al. Exacerbation of heart failure in adiponectin-deficient mice due to impaired regulation of AMPK and glucose metabolism. Cardiovascular Research. 2005;**67**:705-713

[33] Pedersen BK, Febbraio MA. Muscle as an endocrine organ: Focus on muscle-derived interleukin-6. Physiological Reviews. 2008;**88**:1379-1406

[34] Pedersen BKT, Åkerström CA, Nielsen AR, Fischer CP. Role of myokines in exercise and metabolism. Journal of Applied Physiology. 2007;**103**:1093-1098

[35] Shibanuma M, Mashimo J, Mita A, Kuroki T, Nose K. Cloning from a mouse osteoblastic cell line of a set of transforming-growth-factor beta 1-regulated genes, one of which seems to encode a follistatin related polypeptide. European Journal of Biochemistry 1993;**217**:13-19. A. C.

[36] McPherron, Lawler AM Lee SJ. Regulation of skeletal muscle mass in mice by a new TGF-p superfamily member. Nature 1997;**387**:83-90.

[37] Joulia D, Bernardi H, Garandel V, Rabenoelina F, Vernus B, Cabello G. Mechanisms involved in the inhibition of myoblast proliferation and differentiation by myostatin. Experimental Cell Research. 2003;**286**:63-275

[38] Wang M, Yu H, Kim YS, Bidwell CA, Kuang S. Myostatin facilitates slow and inhibits fast myosin heavy chain expression during myogenic differentiation. Biochemical and Biophysical Research Communications. 2012;**426**:83-88

[39] Cleasby ME, Jarmin S, Eilers W, et al. Local overexpression of the myostatin propeptide increases glucose transporter expression and enhances skeletal muscle glucose disposal. The American Journal of Physiology-Endocrinology and Metabolism. 2014;**306**:E814-E823

[40] Allen DL, Cleary AS, Speaker KJ, et al. Myostatin, activin receptor IIb, and follistatin-like-3 gene expression are altered in adipose tissue and skeletal muscle of obese mice. The American Journal of Physiology-Endocrinology and Metabolism. 2008;**294**:E918-E927

[41] Boström WPJ, Jedrychowski MP, et al. A PGC1-α- dependent myokine that drives brown-fat-like development of white fat and thermogenesis. Nature. 2012;**481**:463-468

[42] Lee HJ, Lee JO, Kim N, et al. Irisin, a novel myokine, regulates glucose uptake in skeletal muscle cells via AMPK. Molecular Endocrinology. 2015;**29**:873-881

[43] Seldin MM, Peterson JM, Byerly MS, Wei Z, Wong GW. Myonectin (CTRP15), a novel myokine that links skeletal muscle to systemic lipid homeostasis. Journal of Biological Chemistry. 2012;**287**:11968-11980

[44] Seldin MM, Wong GW. Regulation of tissue crosstalk by skeletal muscle derived myonectin and other myokines. Adipocytes. 2012;**1**:200-202

[45] Cildir G, Akincilar SC, Tergaonkar V. Chronic adipose tissue inflammation: All immune cells on the stage. Trends in Molecular Medicine. 2013;**19**:487-500

[46] Weisberg SP, McCann D, Desai M, Rosenbaum M, Leibel RL, Ferrante AW Jr. Obesity is associated

with macrophage accumulation in adipose tissue. The Journal of Clinical Investigation. 2003;**112**:1796-1808

[47] Xu H, Barnes GT, Yang Q, Tan G, Yang D, Chou CJ, et al. Chronic inflammation in fat plays a crucial role in the development of obesity-related insulin resistance. The Journal of Clinical Investigation. 2003;**112**:1821-1830

[48] Amano SU, Cohen JL, Vangala P, Tencerova M, Nicoloro SM, Yawe JC, et al. Local proliferation of macrophages contributes to obesity-associated adipose tissue inflammation. Cell Metabolism. 2014;**19**:162-171

[49] Hosogai N, Fukuhara A, Oshima K, Miyata Y, Tanaka S, Segawa K, et al. Adipose tissue hypoxia in obesity and its impact on adipocytokine dysregulation. Diabetes. 2007;**56**:901-911

[50] Pasarica M, Rood J, Ravussin E, Schwarz JM, Smith SR, Redman LM. Reduced oxygenation in human obese adipose tissue is associated with impaired insulin suppression of lipolysis. The Journal of Clinical Endocrinology and Metabolism. 2010;**95**:4052-4055

[51] Pasarica M, Sereda OR, Redman LM, Albarado DC, Hymel DT, Roan LE, et al. Reduced adipose tissue oxygenation in human obesity: Evidence for rarefaction, macrophage chemotaxis, and inflammation without an angiogenic response. Diabetes. 2009;**58**:718-725

[52] Ye J, Gao Z, Yin J, He Q. Hypoxia is a potential risk factor for chronic inflammation and adiponectin reduction in adipose tissue of ob/ob and dietary obese mice. American Journal of Physiology. Endocrinology and Metabolism. 2007;**293**:E1118-E1128

Chapter 7

# Roles of Trans and ω Fatty Acids in Health; Special References to Their Differences between Japanese and American Old Men

*Akikazu Takada, Fumiko Shimizu and Shinji Koba*

## Abstract

Omega and trans-fatty acids play important roles in atherogenesis of vascular system. In this review, we discuss such roles in health; there are much differences in coronary heart disease (CHD) rates between the US and Japan. Fatty acids profiles in the plasma are related to risks of CHD. There have been few studies that compared plasma levels of fatty acids, including trans-fatty acids, in people in Japan and the US. Plasma levels of long-chain omega-3 fatty acids (docosahexaenoic acid [DHA] and eicosapentaenoic acid [EPA]) were higher in Japanese men, and omega-6 fatty acids (e.g., arachidonic acid [AA]) were lower compared with American men. American people had higher plasma levels of the major industrially produced trans-fatty acids (IP-TFAs; elaidic and inoelaidic acids), and levels of the potentially cardioprotective, primarily ruminant-derived trans-fatty acid, palmitoelaidic acid (POA) were higher in Japanese men. Plasma levels of saturated or monounsaturated fatty acids were also higher in American men. Only intakes of preference drinks have significant correlation with plasma levels of palmitoelaidic acid and linoelaidic acid. The higher levels of DHA and EPA, along with the lower levels of the IP-TFAs, are consistent with the markedly lower risk for coronary heart disease in Japan vs. the US.

**Keywords:** trans-fatty acids, omega fatty acids, lipid, DHA, EPA, arachidonic acid, palmitoelaidic acid, elaidic acid, linoelaidic acid, food, protein, carbohydrate, preference drink, coffee, tea, cholesterol, GRP120, insulin, GLP-1

## 1. Introduction

Coronary heart disease (CHD) is the leading cause of death worldwide, and certain dietary fatty acids (FAs) are known to play an important role in CHD risk [1]. It has been reported that higher intakes of industrially produced trans-fatty acids (IP-TFA) [2] and of saturated fatty acids (SFAs) are associated with increased risk for CHD [3, 4] and that higher intakes of both the omega-6 (n-6) polyunsaturated fatty acids (PUFAs) and the omega-3 PUFAs are associated with lower risk of CHD [5, 6]. Intakes of the PUFAs (especially the omega-3 class) and IP-TFAs are considered to be biomarkers strongly linked to risks. Because risk for CHD is much lower in Japan than in the US [7], we tried to compare the FA profiles in Japanese and American men over the age of 50.

### 1.1 Configurations of trans-fatty acids and their origins

Trans-fatty acids have at least one double bond in the trans configuration and formed during partial hydrogenation of vegetable oils. This process is used for the conversion of vegetable oils to semisolid fats used for margarines.

Most of trans-fatty acids isomers are monosaturated with carbon number 18 (trans type octadecenoic acid (t-C18:1)). Trans type octadecenoic acids contained in foods are classified 13 isomers depending upon the location of the double bond (**Figure 1**). These trans isomers are produced industrially or naturally. The largest amounts of industrially produced trans-fatty acids are elaidic acids (t 9-C18:1) and those of naturally produced forms are vaccenic acid (t11-C18:1) [8].

In the cis forms of fatty acids, hydrogen atoms are present on the same side of the bond, which causes a bend in the fatty acid chain, whereas the trans form has hydrogen atoms in the opposite sides of the chain, which straightens the fatty acid chain (upper figure). There are many isomers in carbon 18 fatty acids. Elaidic acid has the double bond at the ninth carbon atom (t9-18:1). Oleic acid has the double bond at the same location (c9-18:1). Partially hydrogenated oils contain mixture of isomers in which the trans form may be detected anywhere between the 4th and 14th carbon. Smaller amounts of isomers with a second trans double bond (trans,trans-18:2) are also present.

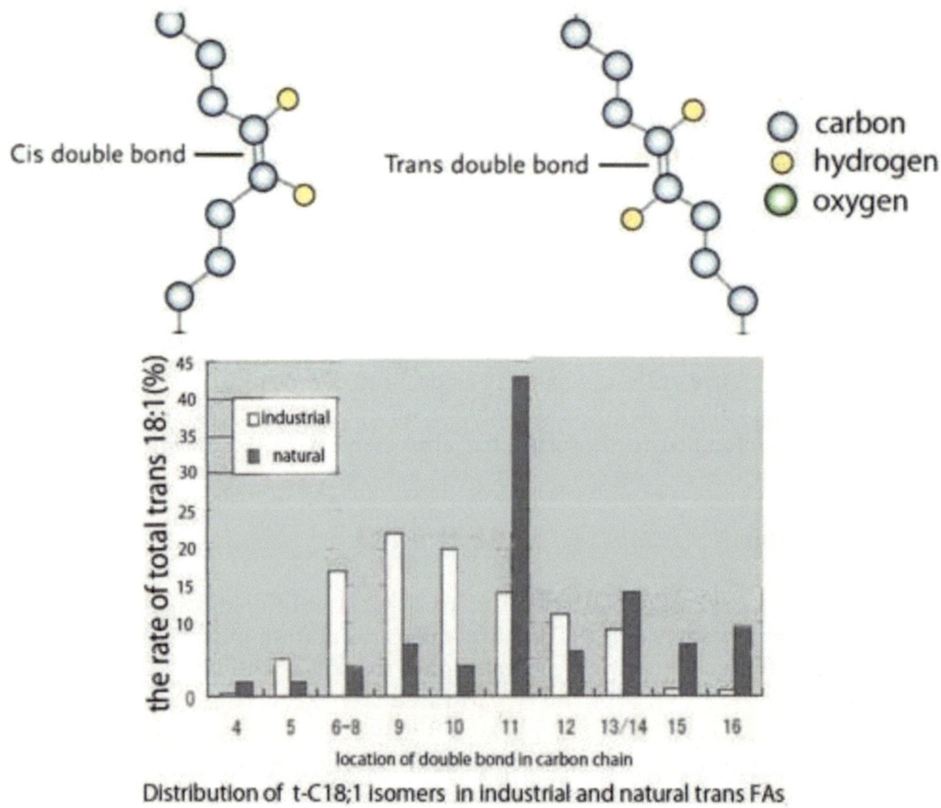


**Figure 1.**
*The configuration of cis and trans forms of the double bond.*

### 1.2 Molecular mechanisms of trans-fatty acids

Fatty acids modulate cell functions. They change membrane fluidity and responses of membrane receptors. Fatty acids not only bind to membrane receptors but also bind to and modulate nuclear receptors that regulate gene transcription, peroxisome-proliferator-activated receptors, liver X receptor, and sterol regulatory element-binding protein 1 [9] (**Figure 2**). Fatty acids modulate metabolic and inflammatory responses of the endoplasmic reticulum [10].

Trans-fatty acids change the secretion, lipid composition, and the size of apoB100 produced by hepatic cells [11, 12]. In hepatocytes, trans-fatty acids increase the accumulation and secretion of free cholesterol and cholesterol esters [11]. Trans-fatty acids increase plasma activity of cholesteryl ester transfer protein [13], which may result in decreases in plasma levels of high density lipoprotein (HDL) and increase in the levels of low density lipoprotein (LDL) and very low density lipoprotein (VLDL).

Trans-fatty acids modulate monocyte and macrophage functions resulting in increase in the production of tissue necrosis factor (TNF)-α and interleukin-6 [14]. Endothelial dysfunctions are caused by trans-fatty acids, and arterial dilatation is impaired due to nitric oxide [15].

Fatty acid metabolism of adipocytes was affected by trans-fatty acids, causing reduced triglyceride uptake, reduced esterification of cholesterol, and increased production of free fatty acids [16]. In animal studies, the gene expression was changed by the consumption of trans-fatty acids in adipocytes. These gene products are peroxisome-proliferator-activated receptor-γ, resistin, and lipoprotein lipase [17].

Trans-fatty acids may affect plasma lipid levels due to changes in hepatocytes of the production, secretion, and catabolism of lipoproteins and plasma levels of

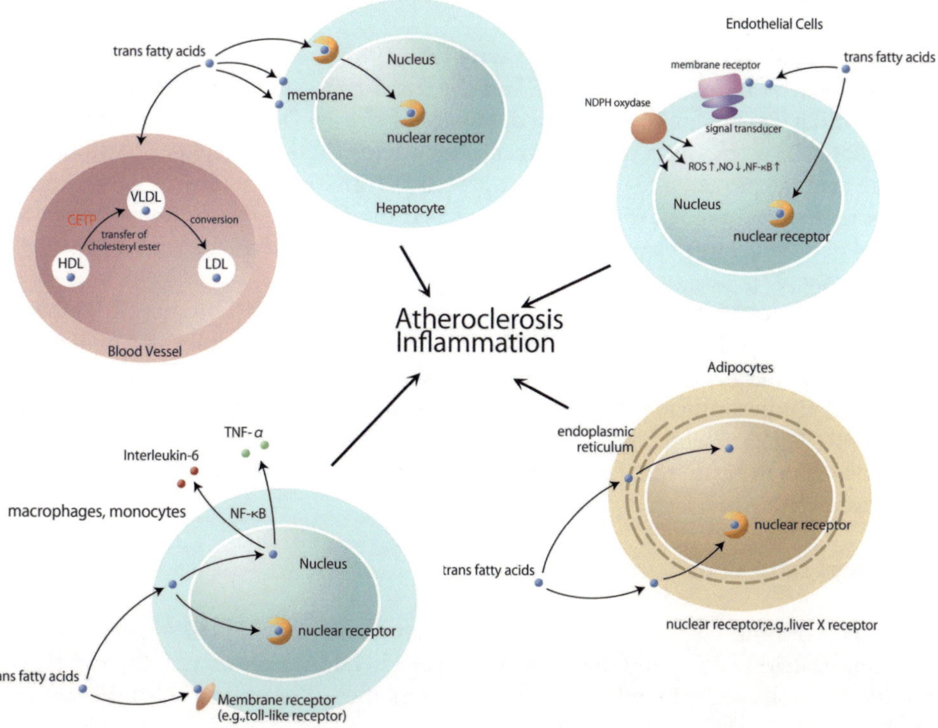


**Figure 2.**
*Effects of trans-fatty acids.*

cholesteryl ester transfer protein (CETP) (upper left panel). In adipocytes, trans-fatty acids change fatty acid metabolism and, possibly, inflammatory responses. When trans fats are taken, nitric acid-dependent endothelial dysfunction is observed and circulating adhesion molecules increase. Trans fat modulates monocyte and macrophage function (lower left panel). Membrane receptors may affect subcellular mechanisms. These receptors localize with and are influenced by specific membrane phospholipids (upper right panel) such as endothelia nitric oxide synthetase or toll-like receptors. Trans-fatty acids may bind to nuclear receptors-regulating gene transcription such as liver X receptor (lower left panel).

### 1.3 Effects on cardiovascular diseases

Trans-fatty acids may increase the risks of coronary heart disease (CHD). In a meta-analysis of four prospective cohort studies, a 2% increase in energy intake from trans-fatty acids was shown to be associated with a 23% increase in the incidence of CHD [18–21].

There are many papers showing increased risks of CHD in patients with high fatty acids levels [22–25]. These data are obtained using cohorts of Western populations.

Koba et al. [26] recently reported using Japanese adult males that total trans-fatty acids levels were similar between acute coronary syndrome (ACS) and control subjects. Palmitelaidic acid levels were lower in ACS patients and were significantly directly associated with HDL cholesterol (HDL-C) and n-3 polyunsaturated FA (n-3 PUFA). Linoleic trans isomers (total C18:2 TFA) and primary industrially produced TFA (IP-TFAs) were significantly higher in ACS patients. Total trans-C18:1 isomers were comparable between ACS and control.

### 1.4 Intakes of trans-fatty acids in people of US and Japan

Allison et al. [27] used food intake data from1989 to 1991 Continuing Survey of Food Intakes by Individuals (CSFII) and the trans-fatty acid contents of specific foods, which were calculated from a data base of the US Department of Agriculture. These data show the mean levels of trans-fatty acids intakes of US population.

The average percentage of energy ingested as trans-fatty acids was 2.6%, and the average percentage of total fat ingested as trans-fatty acids was 7.4%. Across all age and gender groups examined, estimates ranged from 2.6 to 2.8% and 7.1 to 7.9%, respectively [27].

In Japan, mean total fat and trans-fatty acid intake was 56.9 g/day (27.7% total energy) and 1.7 g/day (0.8% total energy), respectively, for women and 66.8 g/day (25.5% total energy) and 1.7 g/day (0.7% total energy) for men [28].

Recent studies indicate that the average trans-fatty acids intake was estimated to be 0.92–0.96 g/day, which was 0.44–0.47% of total daily energy intakes [29].

These data indicate that Japanese take far less amounts of trans-fatty acids compared with American.

### 1.5 Omega fatty acids

Intakes of long-chain ω-3 fatty acids (eicosapentaenoic acid (EPA), docosa pentaenoic acid (DPA), and docosahexanoic acid (DHA)) found in fish, and fish oils has been shown to be related to the low incidence of coronary heart disease in the Inuit people of Greenland [30].

We do not review roles of such fatty acids in health and disease in details.

**Figure 3** summarizes roles of EPA in causing various dysfunctions of the body.

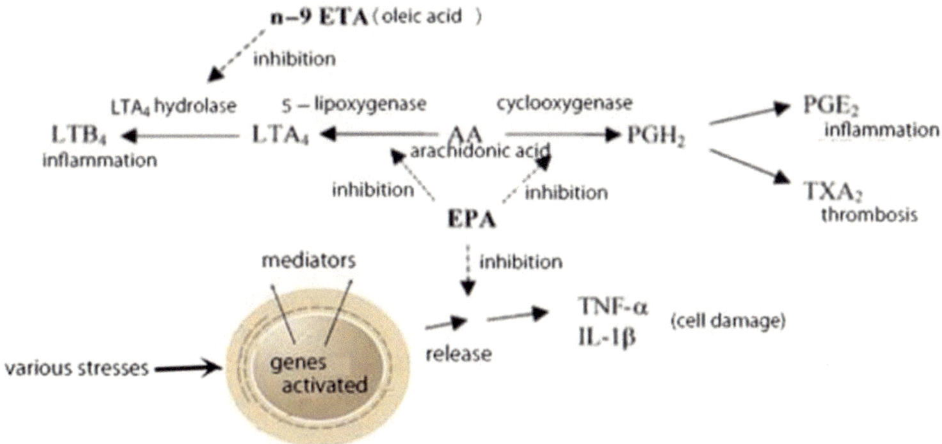


**Figure 3.**
*Roles of EPA in the prevention of cell damage, inflammation, or thrombosis.*

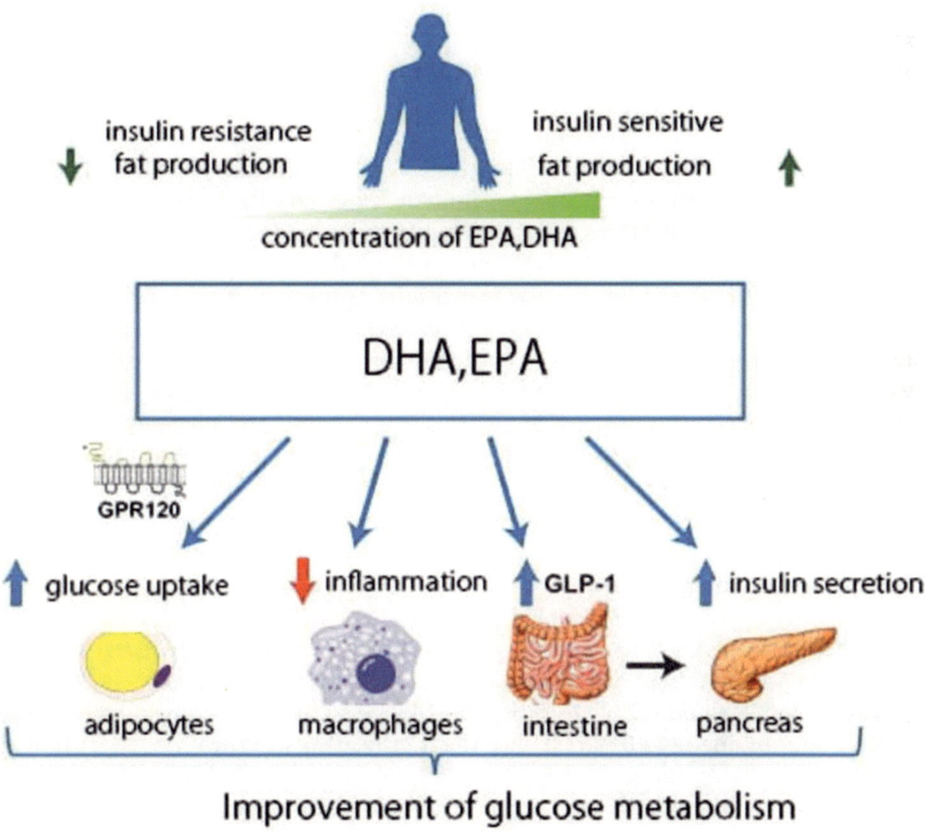


**Figure 4.**
*Function of G-protein-coupled receptor 120 as a receptor of DHA and EPA.*

Arachidonic acid (n-6 polyunsaturated fatty acid "PUFA") is converted to PGH2 (prostaglandin $H_2$, which is converted to prostaglandin $E_2$, inflammatory mediator) or to $TXA_2$ (thromboxane $A_2$), causing thrombosis. AA is also converted to $LTA_4$ (leukotriene $A_2$), then to leukotriene $B_4$, inflammatory mediator [31].

Cells produce TNF-α or interleukin (IL)-1β, which case cell damages.

EPA inhibits such processes, preventing cell damages, inflammation, and thrombosis. DHA may work in the similar ways as EPA.

### 1.6 ω fatty acid receptor

GPR120 is proposed to function as an ω-3 FA receptor/sensor in pro-inflammatory macrophages and mature adipocytes. By signaling through GPR120, DHA and EPA mediate potent anti-inflammatory effects to inhibit both TLR (toll-like receptor) and TNF-α inflammatory signaling pathways [32].

DHA and EPA stimulate GRP 120 and cause a decrease of glucose uptake by adipocytes, inhibit inflammation by macrophages, secrete glucagon-like peptide 1 (GLP-1), and increase insulin secretion by pancreas (**Figure 4**).

These data suggest that DHA and EPA may be effective for prevention and treatment of cardiovascular disease and diabetes mellitus.

## 2. Differences of plasma levels of fatty acids between Japanese and American old men

### 2.1 Materials and methods

#### *2.1.1 Participants*

In Japan, we recruited 44 male volunteers older than 50. They were friends and family members of the research team for this study [33, 34]. Exclusion criteria included the use of medications to treat diabetes, hyperlipidemia, hypertension, and/or cardiovascular disease (CVD). Smokers were also excluded. The 76 US men were participants in the Chicago Area Sleep Study, a prospective cohort study to examine risk factors for the development of sleep disorders [35]. This cohort excluded men with known sleep disturbances but did not exclude for the chronic conditions excluded in the Japanese cohort. We collected blood samples after an overnight fast, and plasma was isolated for fatty acid analysis. We obtained an informed consent prior to conducting the protocol which had been approved by the Ethical Committee of Showa Women's University and Saiseikai Shibuya Satellite Clinic. The Chicago Area Sleep Study was approved by the Northwestern University Institutional Review Board.

### 2.2 Analyses of plasma samples

Fatty acids levels were measured in plasma obtained from ethylenediamine tetraacetic acid anticoagulated blood samples. Samples were frozen at −80°C until analyzed at Omegaquant, LLC (Sioux Falls, SD, USA). After thawing, an aliquot of plasma was combined (1.40 parts) with the methylating mixture (boron trifluoride in methanol [14%], toluene, and methanol [35/30/35, vv]), shaken at 100°C for 45 min. After cooling, 40 parts of both hexane and distilled water were added. After briefly vortexing, the samples were spun to separate layers, and an aliquot of the hexane layer that contained the fatty acid methyl esters was analyzed by gas chromatography as previously described.

### 2.3 Statistical analysis

Student's t test was used for the comparison of two groups, and $p < 0.05$ was considered as significant difference. Results are expressed as mean ± SD. Spearman's correlation tests were used to examine statistical significance.

## 3. Results

The ages of the two cohorts was reasonably similar (Japan, 61 ± 10 and US, 57 ± 5 years), as were the body mass indexes (24.9 ± 3.7 vs. 25.1 ± 3.4 kg/m$^2$) (**Figure 5**).

Of the fatty acids that constituted at least 1% of the total in either cohorts, those that are significantly higher in Japanese men than US men were as follows: palmitic, palmitoleic, arachidic, EPA, and DHA. Those that were lower in the Japanese men were as follows: linoleic acid (LA), dihomo-gamma linolenic acid (DGLA), and AA (**Table 1**).

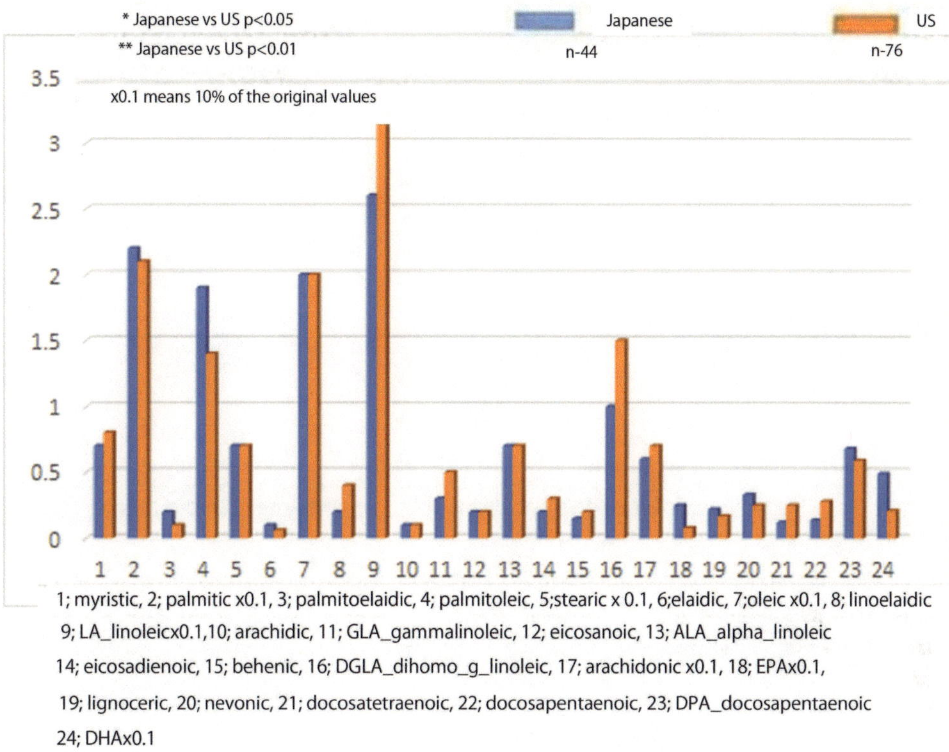


**Figure 5.**
*Profiles of plasma levels of fatty acids of Japanese and American old men.*

| | Japanese (n = 44) | American (n = 76) |
|---|---|---|
| Age | 62.4 ± 9.6 | 57.5 ± 4.3 |
| Height (m) | 1.68 ± 0.07 | 1.70 ± 0.1 |
| Weight (kg) | 68.8 ± 10.9 | 74.4 ± 12.1 |
| Body mass index (BMI) | 24.3 ± 3.2 | 25.3 ± 3.4 |
| Total cholesterol (mg/dL) | 209.9 ± 32.3 | 185 ± 33.5 |
| Triglyceride (mg/dL) | 126.4 ± 81.3 | 118.0 ± 62.8 |
| HDL-C (mg/dL) | 60.9 ± 16.6 | 54.0 ± 15.7 |
| LDL-C (mg/dL) | 123.8 ± 30.2 | 107.0 ± 29.6 |
| Fasting blood glucose (mg/dL) | 91.7 ± 16.3 | 97 ± 22.3 |

**Table 1.**
*Backgrounds of various parameters of healthy old men in Japan and US.*

**Figure 6** compares plasma levels of palmitoelaidic, elaidic, and linoelaidic acids. IP-TFAs (elaidic and mainly industrially produced linoelaidic), although of low abundance in both cohorts, were considerably higher in the US than in Japan. Palmitoleic was slightly but significantly higher in Japan (**Figure 7**).

Plasma levels of DHA and EPA are higher in Japanese than American old men; on the other hand, plasma levels of arachidonic acid and dihomoγlinoleinic acid are higher in American than Japanese old men.

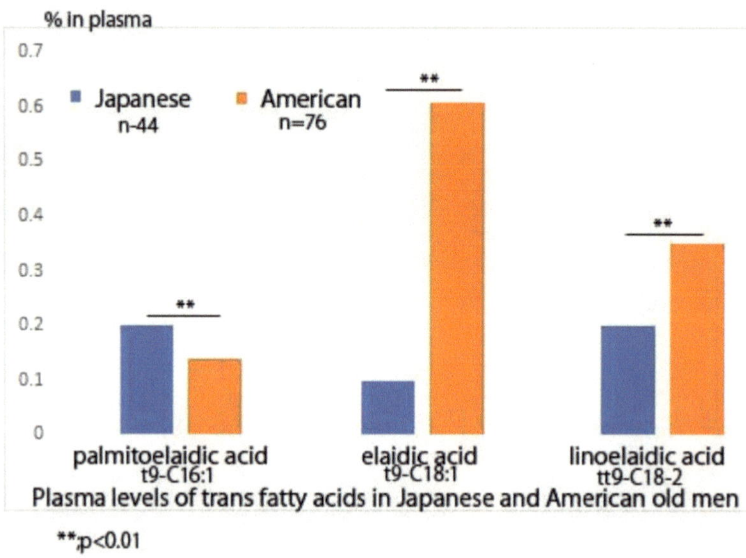


**Figure 6.**
*Plasma levels of trans-fatty acids in Japanese and American old men.*

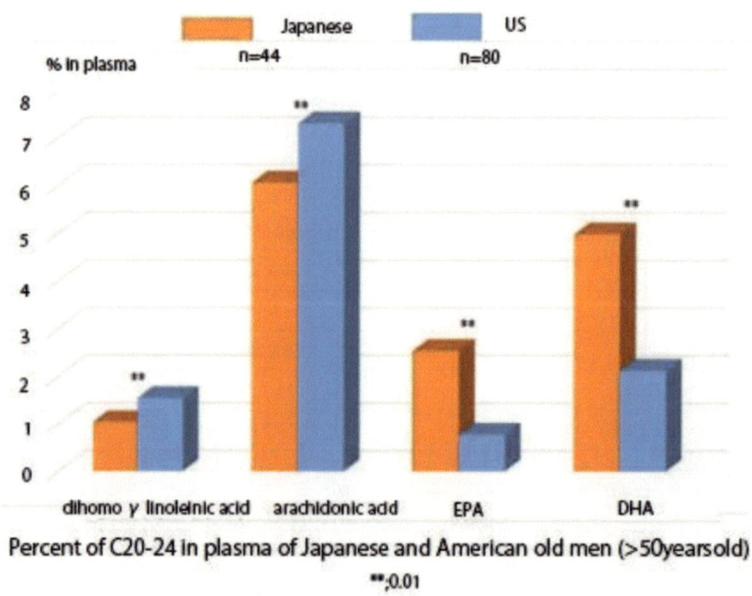


**Figure 7.**
*Comparison of plasma levels of C20–22 fatty acids between Japanese and American old men.*

| Plasma fatty acids (% of total) | Japanese (n = 44) | US (n = 76) | ss |
|---|---|---|---|
| Myristic | 0.7 ± 0.2 | 0.85 ± 0.34 | ** |
| Palmitic | 22.3 ± 1.3 | 21.23 ± 2.13 | * |
| Palmitoelaidic (trans) | 0.2 ± 0.1 | 0.14 ± 0.07 | ** |
| Palmitoleic | 1.9 ± 0.6 | 1.45 ± 0.80 | ** |
| Stearic | 7.0 ± 0.7 | 7.24 ± 0.83 | |
| Elaidic (trans) | 0.1 ± 0.01 | 0.61 ± 0.34 | ** |
| Oleic | 20.0 ± 2.6 | 19.96 ± 3.34 | |
| Linoelaidic (trans) | 0.2 ± 0.1 | 0.35 ± 0.12 | ** |
| Linoleic (LA) | 26.3 ± 4.0 | 32.83 ± 5.24 | ** |
| Arachidic | 0.13 ± 0.04 | 0.13 ± 0.04 | |
| Gamma linolenic | 0.3 ± 0.1 | 0.53 ± 0.27 | ** |
| Eicosenoic | 0.2 ± 0.04 | 0.15 ± 0.05 | |
| Alpha-linolenic | 0.7 ± 0.2 | 0.72 ± 0.32 | |
| Eicosadienoic | 0.2 ± 0.03 | 0.29 ± 0.07 | ** |
| Behenic | 0.15 ± 0.02 | 0.20 ± 0.10 | ** |
| Dihomo-gamma linolenic (DGLA) | 1.0 ± 0.2 | 1.56 ± 0.37 | ** |
| Arachidonic (AA) | 6.0 ± 1.1 | 7.38 ± 2.18 | ** |
| Eicosapentaenoic (EPA) | 2.5 ± 1.3 | 0.77 ± 0.60 | ** |
| Lignoceric | 0.22 ± 0.10 | 0.18 ± 0.07 | * |
| Nervonic | 0.33 ± 0.18 | 0.26 ± 0.10 | * |
| Docosatetraenoic | 0.12 ± 0.04 | 0.26 ± 0.11 | ** |
| Docosapentaenoic (n6) | 0.14 ± 0.04 | 0.18 ± 0.08 | ** |
| Docosapentaenoic (n3) | 0.68 ± 0.26 | 0.59 ± 0.14 | * |
| Docosahexaenoic (DHA) | 5.0 ± 1.5 | 2.14 ± 0.85 | ** |

*ss, statistical significance.*
*$^{*}p < 0.05$.*
*$^{**}p < 0.01$.*

**Table 2.**
*Comparison of fatty acids profiles between Japanese and American men.*

**Table 2** summarizes plasma levels of important fatty acids between Japanese and American men.

## 4. Food intakes and plasma levels of fatty acids

Participants were given self-administered diet history questionnaires and described answers on each item by recollection of diets they took (7 days dietary recall). We used a brief-type self-administered diet history questionnaire (BDHQ) by using which the Japanese Ministry of Health, Labour and Welfare reports National Nutrition Surveys. From these questionnaires, we calculated the intakes of energy and varieties of foods such as proteins, carbohydrates, lipids vitamins, etc.

### 4.1 Results

**Table 3** shows that only preference drinks such as tea and coffee had significant correlations with plasma levels of palmitoelaidic acid and linoelaidic acid.

| | Palmitelaidic | Elaidic | Linoelaidic |
|---|---|---|---|
| Energy | 0.319 | −0.135 | 0.181 |
| Protein | 0.239 | 0.031 | 0.034 |
| Animal protein | 0.233 | 0.135 | 0.034 |
| Vegetable protein | 0.193 | −0.081 | 0.152 |
| Lipid | 0.187 | 0.120 | 0.034 |
| Animal lipid | 0.188 | 0.154 | 0.094 |
| Vegetable lipid | 0.167 | 0.027 | −0.066 |
| Carbohydrate | 0.188 | −0.197 | 0.138 |
| Na | 0.128 | 0.033 | −0.073 |
| K | 0.223 | −0.015 | 0.137 |
| Ca | 0.099 | 0.263 | −0.021 |
| Mg | 0.283 | −0.003 | 0.143 |
| Phosphorus | 0.230 | 0.088 | 0.020 |
| Iron | 0.193 | −0.120 | 0.112 |
| Zinc | 0.109 | 0.081 | 0.072 |
| Copper | 0.211 | −0.066 | 0.163 |
| Mn | 0.422 | −0.059 | 0.113 |
| Retinol | 0.307 | −0.195 | 0.054 |
| β-Carotene | −0.001 | −0.049 | −0.005 |
| Vit D | 0.295 | −0.001 | −0.066 |
| Tocopherol | 0.167 | −0.049 | −0.004 |
| Vit K | 0.098 | 0.014 | 0.083 |
| Vit B1 | 0.095 | 0.119 | 0.098 |
| Vit B2 | 0.246 | 0.169 | 0.135 |
| Niacine | 0.320 | −0.012 | 0.081 |
| Vit B6 | 0.239 | −0.036 | 0.129 |
| Vit B12 | 0.353 | −0.090 | 0.049 |
| Folic acid | 0.333 | −0.120 | 0.080 |
| Pantothenic acid | 0.299 | 0.120 | 0.083 |
| Vit C | 0.214 | −0.040 | 0.034 |
| Saturated fatty acids | 0.209 | 0.144 | 0.112 |
| Monovalent fatty acids | 0.156 | 0.126 | −0.004 |
| Multivalent fatty acids | 0.179 | 0.024 | −0.062 |
| Cholesterol | 0.221 | −0.025 | 0.125 |
| Soluble dietary fiber | 0.133 | −0.080 | 0.155 |
| Insoluble dietary fiber | 0.125 | −0.047 | 0.076 |
| Total dietary fiber | 0.082 | 0.027 | 0.089 |
| Salt | 0.128 | 0.033 | −0.073 |
| Preference drinks | 0.586** | −0.263 | 0.511* |

*Mean ± SD.*
*$^{*}p < 0.05$.*
*$^{**}p < 0.01$.*

**Table 3.**
*Correlations between foods intake and plasma levels of fatty acids.*

## 5. Discussion

Fatty acids are major components of blood vessels. So their changes exert tremendous impact to pathophysiology of cardiovascular system.

Epidemiological studies repeatedly showed that Japanese people had lower incidence of CVD, compared with American people [7]. As discussed below, kinds of intaken foods, life-styles, and genetics may contribute to such differences.

We thought the measurements of fatty acids composition in plasma may help to elucidate such differences between Japanese and American people.

We compared plasma levels of fatty acids between Japanese and American men over 50 years of age. We found, not surprisingly, that levels of EPA and DHA are higher in Japanese than American and that levels of arachidonic acid are lower in Japanese. Although both Japanese and American take meat, egg, and fish, fish has far more omega-3 fatty acids compared to eggs. When we eat larger amounts of omega-3 fatty acids such as DHA and EPA, omega-3 fatty acids are known to replace omega-6 fatty acids in cell membrane [36]. The omega-3 fatty acids are found predominantly in oily fish, whereas arachidonic acid (the major long chain omega-6 fatty acid) is contained in meats and eggs and can be synthesized (albeit very slowly) [37]. The differences between Japanese and US men in regard to the consumption of these types of foods can help explain these differences in blood levels [38]. The other major finding of this study was the lower levels of IP-TFA such as linoelaidic acid in Japanese vs. the US men.

Currently, CHD death rates in Japan are 3× lower for women and 4× lower for men (ages 35–74) compared with the US. Among 30 countries for which the American Heart Association provided CHD death rates in its 2017 Statistical Update [7], Japan had the second and third lowest rates (men and women, respectively) compared with the US. Sekikawa et al. [39] showed in 2014 that the calcification of the coronary artery was twice in American compared with Japanese men, but the calcification of Hawaiian Japanese was similar to that of people on the US mainland.

These results do not necessarily prove differences of CVD incidences between Japanese and American are due to foods and lifestyle. Since Japanese immigrants to the US have increased CHD mortality [40], although still lower US Whites, it appears that some genetic variabilities between American and Japanese must be responsible for this difference. However, the possibility that differences in dietary fatty acid patterns may contribute to this phenomenon is the subject of this report.

We found that the levels of the long-chain omega-3 fatty acids such as EPA and DHA were 2–3× higher in Japan vs. the US. The relationship of fish and dietary omega-3 fatty acids and cardiovascular disease (CVD) has been investigated in numerous studies and comprehensive reviews and recommendations exist. Still controversies exist. A recent meta-analysis of randomized trials with omega-3 fatty acids [41] did not find a statistically significant reduction in CVD mortality, but in these researches, some important factors were said to be ignored [42–44]. Other systematic reviews have reported mortality benefits for omega-3 fatty acids [45, 46], and omega-3 biomarker levels have been strongly associated with risk for fatal CHD in still other meta-analyses [47, 48]. Hence, higher omega-3 levels could at least partly explain the lower CHD risk in Japan.

We also found that IP-trans-fatty acid such as linoelaidic acid was lower in Japan than US. The reported intake of IP-TFA is 75% lower in Japan than in the US, again supporting the observed differences in biomarker levels. Circulating 18:2 trans-fatty acids was shown to be most adversely associated with total mortality, mainly due to the increased risk of CVD [23]. It was also positively associated with total mortality and CHD.

It may be surprising that TFA is not necessarily adverse for health. Some are beneficial for health. In a recent study from Germany, total trans-fatty acids in erythrocyte membranes were shown to be inversely associated with mortality, but this was mainly driven by the naturally occurring 16:1 trans (trans-palmitoleic acid) [49]. As to relationship between IP-TFA or SFA intakes and CHD mortality, excessive intakes of both had a greater impact on risk for CHD in the US compared with Japan, whereas insufficient intakes of omega-6 PUFAs had about the same impact on risk in both countries [50].

Our results also indicate that plasma levels of SFAs are higher in American than in Japanese. Saturated fatty acids are considered to be one of the dietary risk factors of CVD, primarily because these fats raise LDL-cholesterol levels. Many health and government organizations have recommended the reduction of intakes of SFA s to lower the incidence of CVD. Although this difference in SFA plasma levels may also be one of the reasons that Americans have a higher mortality rate for CVD than Japanese, plasma saturated (and monounsaturated) fatty acids are claimed to be relatively poor markers of dietary SFA (saturated fatty acid) intake [51].

Plasma fatty acid profiles in older men from Japan and US differed in many ways that are consistent with the lower rate of CHD in the former country. Efforts to lower TFA levels and increase EPA + DHA levels may help lower risk for CHD in the US, and current trends in Japan toward a more western diet [52] should be discouraged.

As to relationship between TFA or SFA intakes and CHD mortality, excessive intakes of both had a greater impact on risk for CHD in the US compared with Japan, whereas insufficient intakes of omega-6 PUFAs had about the same impact on risk in both countries [50]. As stated above, naturally occurring trans fats are consumed in smaller amounts (about 0.5% of total energy intake) in meats and dairy products from cows, sheep, and other ruminants; these trans fats are produced by the action of bacteria in the ruminant stomach [22]. Since trans-fatty acids are not used in foods in Japan, all the trans-fatty acids must come from meat or dairy products. We found that there was no relationship between various foods intake and plasma levels of trans-fatty acids in Japanese old men. Only intakes of preference drinks such as tea and coffee had significant relationship with plasma levels of palmitoelaidic acid and linoelaidic acid. These results seem to indicate that plasma levels of trans-fatty acids are not derived from foods but derived by intestinal microbes.

Human gut microbes are important in neural, endocrine, and immune communication with the host [53]. Communication is considered to be bidirectional. Mediators of microbiota-gut-brain communication affected by microbial metabolism include short-chain fatty acids, neurotransmitters such as serotonin, γ-aminobutyric acid (GABA), hormones such as cortisol, and immune system mediators such as quinolinic acid [51].

In conclusion, some of trans-fatty acids may be produced by hydrogenation of fatty acids by gut microbes.

## 6. Conclusion

We here report our results of comparison of plasma levels of fatty acids between healthy old men in Japan and the US.

The higher levels of DHA and EPA, along with the lower levels of the IP-TFAs, are consistent with the markedly lower risk for coronary heart disease in Japan vs. the US.

Various foods intake may not affect plasma levels of trans-fatty acids in Japanese old men except for preference drinks such as tea or coffee.

The higher levels of DHA and EPA, along with the lower levels of the IP-TFAs, are consistent with the markedly lower risk for coronary heart disease in Japan vs. the US.

Our results also indicate that plasma levels of SFAs are higher in American than in Japanese. Saturated fatty acids are considered to be one of the dietary risk factors of CVD, primarily because these fats raise LDL-cholesterol levels.

## Acknowledgements

Experiments were designed and performed by all of the authors. AT and WSH wrote the manuscript. Statistical analyses were done by FS. All authors read the manuscript and approved the final version. All the authors take responsibility for the final content.

## Author details

Akikazu Takada[1*], Fumiko Shimizu[2] and Shinji Koba[3]

1 Hamamatsu University School of Medicine, Tokyo, Japan

2 Faculty of Life and Environmental Sciences, Showa Women's University, Tokyo, Japan

3 Division of Cardiology, Department of Medicine, Showa University School of Medicine, Tokyo, Japan

*Address all correspondence to: takadaa@mwd.biglobe.ne.jp

## References


[1] Lim SS, Vos T, Flaxman AD, et al. A comparative risk assessment of burden of disease and injury attributable to 67 risk factors and risk factor clusters in 21 regions, 1990-2010: A systematic analysis for the Global Burden of Disease Study 2010. Lancet. 2012;**380**:2224-2260. DOI: 10.1016/S0140-6736(12)61766-8

[2] Mozaffarian D, Willett WC. Trans fatty acids and cardiovascular risk: A unique cardiometabolic imprint? Current Atherosclerosis Reports. 2007;**9**:486-493

[3] Mozaffarian D, Micha R, Wallace S. Effects on coronary heart disease of increasing polyunsaturated fat in place of saturated fat: A systematic review and meta-analysis of randomized controlled trials. PLoS Medicine. 2010;7:e1000252. DOI: 10.1371/journal.pmed.1000252

[4] Jakobsen MU, O'Reilly EJ, Heitmann BL, Pereira MA, Bälter K, Fraser GE, et al. Major types of dietary fat and risk of coronary heart disease: A pooled analysis of 11 cohort studies. American Journal of Clinical Nutrition. 2009;**89**:1425-1432. DOI: 10.3945/ajcn.2008.27124

[5] Farvid MS, Ding M, Pan A, Sun Q, Chiuve SE, Steffen LM, et al. Dietary linoleic acid and risk of coronary heart disease: A systematic review and meta-analysis of prospective cohort studies. Circulation. 2014;**130**:1568-1578. DOI: 10.1161/CIRCULATIONAHA.114.010236

[6] Chowdhury R, Warnakula S, Kunutsor S, Crowe F, Ward HA, Johnson L, et al. Association of dietary, circulating, and supplement fatty acids with coronary risk: A systematic review and meta-analysis. Annals of Internal Medicine. 2014;**160**:398-406. DOI: 10.7326/M13-1788

[7] Benjamin EJ, Blaha MJ, Chiuve SE, et al. Heart disease and stroke statistics-2017 update: A report from the American Heart Association. Circulation. 2017;**135**:e146-e603. DOI: 10.1161/CIR.0000000000000485

[8] Wolff RL, Combe NA, Destaillats F, Boué C, Precht D, Molkentin J, et al. Follow-up of the delta4 to delta16 trans-18:1 isomer profile and content in French processed foods containing partially hydrogenated vegetable oils during the period 1995-1999. Analytical and nutritional implications. Lipids. 2000;**35**:815-825. DOI: 10.1007/s11745-000-0590-2

[9] Vanden Heuvel JP. Diet, fatty acids, and regulation of genes important for heart disease. Current Atherosclerosis Reports. 2004;**6**:432-440

[10] Hotamisligil GS. Role of endoplasmic reticulum stress and c-Jun NH2-terminal kinase pathways in inflammation and origin of obesity and diaabetes. Diabetes. 2005;**54** (Suppl 2):S73-S78. DOI: 10.2337/diabetes.54.suppl_2.s73

[11] Dashti N, Feng Q, Freeman MR, Gandhi M, Franklin FA. Trans polyunsaturated fatty acids have more adverse effects than saturated fatty acids on the concentration and composition of lipoproteins secreted by human hepatoma HepG2 cells. The Journal of Nutrition. 2002;**132**:2651-2659. DOI: 10.1093/jn/132.9.2651

[12] Mitmesser SH, Carr TP. Trans fatty acids alter the lipid composition and size of apoB-100-containing lipoproteins secreted by HepG2 cells. The Journal of Nutritional Biochemistry. 2005;**16**:178-183. DOI: 10.1016/j.jnutbio.2004.11.004

[13] van Tol A, Zock PL, van Gent T, Scheek LM, Katan MB. Dietary

trans fatty acids increase serum cholesterylester transfer protein activity in man. Atherosclerosis. 1995;**115**:129-134. DOI: 10.1016/0021-9150(94)05509-h

[14] Han SN, Leka LS, Lichtenstein AH, Ausman LM, Schaefer EJ, Meydani SN. Effect of hydrogenated and saturated, relative to polyunsaturated, fat on immune and inflammatory responses of adults with moderate hypercholesterolemia. Journal of Lipid Research. 2002;**43**:445-452. Available from: http://www.jlr.org/content/43/3/445.long

[15] de Roos NM, Bots ML, Katan MB. Replacement of dietary saturated fatty acids by trans fatty acids lowers serum HDL cholesterol and impairs endothelial function in healthy men and women. Arteriosclerosis, Thrombosis, and Vascular Biology. 2001;**21**:1233-1237

[16] Matthan NR, Cianflone K, Lichtenstein AH, Ausman LM, Jauhiainen M, Jones PJ. Hydrogenated fat consumption affects acylation-stimulating protein levels and cholesterol esterification rates in moderately hypercholesterolemic women. Journal of Lipid Research. 2001;**42**:1841-1848. Available from: http://www.jlr.org/content/42/11/1841.long

[17] Saravanan N, Haseeb A, Ehtesham NZ, Ghafoorunissa X. Differential effects of dietary saturated and trans-fatty acids on expression of genes associated with insulin sensitivity in rat adipose tissue. European Journal of Endocrinology. 2005;**153**:159-165. DOI: 10.1530/eje.1.01946

[18] Pietinen P, Ascherio A, Korhonen P, Hartman AM, Willett WC, Albanes D, et al. Intake of fatty acids and risk of coronary heart disease in a cohort of Finnish men: The Alpha-Tocopherol, Beta-Carotene Cancer Prevention Study. American Journal of Epidemiology. 1997;**145**:876-887. DOI: 10.1093/oxfordjournals.aje.a009047

[19] Oomen CM, Ocke MC, Feskens EJ, van Erp-Baart MA, Kok FJ, Kromhout D. Association between trans fatty acid intake and 10-year risk of coronary heart disease in the Zutphen Elderly Study: A prospective population-based study. Lancet. 2001;**357**:746-751. DOI: 10.1016/s0140-6736(00)04166-0

[20] Oh K, Hu FB, Manson JE, Stampfer MJ, Willett WC. Dietary fat intake and risk of coronary heart disease in women: 20 years of follow-up of the Nurses' Health Study. American Journal of Epidemiology. 2005;**161**:672-679. DOI: 10.1093/aje/kwi085

[21] Ascherio A, Rimm EB, Giovannucci EL, Spiegelman D, Stampfer M, Willett WC. Dietary fat and risk of coronary heart disease in men: Cohort follow up study in the United States. BMJ. 1996;**313**:84-90. DOI: 10.1136/bmj.313.7049.84

[22] Mozaffarian D, Katan MB, Ascherio A, Stampfer MJ, Willett WC. Trans fatty acids and cardiovascular disease. New England Journal of Medicine. 2006;**354**:1601-1613. DOI: 10.1136/bmj.313.7049.84

[23] Lemaitre RN, King IB, Mozaffarian D, Kuller LH, Tracy RP, Siscovick DS. Plasma phospholipid trans fatty acids, fatal ischemic heart disease, and sudden cardiac death in older adults: The Cardiovascular Health Study. Circulation. 2006;**114**:209-215. DOI: 10.1161/CIRCULATIONAHA.106.620336

[24] Sun Q, Ma J, Campos H, Hankinson SE, Manson JE, Stampfer MJ, et al. A prospective study of trans fatty acids in erythrocytes and risk of coronary heart disease. Circulation.

2007;**115**:1858-1865. DOI: 10.1161/CIRCULATIONAHA.106.679985

[25] Wang Q, Imamura F, Lemaitre RN, Rimm EB, Wang W, King IB, et al. Plasma phospholipid trans-fatty acids levels, cardiovascular diseases, and total mortality: The Cardiovascular Health Study. Journal of the American Heart Association. 2014;**3**(4). pii: e000914. DOI: 10.1161/JAHA.114.000914

[26] Koba S, Takao T, Shimizu F, Ogawa M, Ishii Y, Yokota Y, et al. Comparison of plasma levels of different species of trans fatty acids in Japanese male patients with acute coronary yndrome versus healthy men. Atherosclerosis. 2019;**284**:173-180. DOI: 10.1016/j.atherosclerosis.2019.02.025

[27] Allison DB, Egan SK, Barraj LM, Caughman C, Infante M, Heimbach JT. Estimated intakes of trans fatty and other fatty acids in the US population. Journal of the American Dietetic Association. 1999;**99**:166-174. DOI: 10.1016/S0002-8223(99)00041-3

[28] Yamada M, Sasaki S, Murakami K, Takahashi Y, Okubo H, Hirota N, et al. Estimation of caffeine intake in Japanese adults using 16 d weighed diet records based on a food composition database newly developed for Japanese populations. Public Health Nutrition. 2010;**13**:663-672. DOI: 10.1017/S1368980009992023

[29] Available from: www.maff.go.jp/j/syouan/seisaku/papers_posters/pdf/47th

[30] Bang HO, Dyerberg J. Plasma lipids and lipoproteins in Greenlandic west coast Eskimos. Acta Medica Scandinavica. 1972;**192**:85-94. DOI: 10.1111/j.0954-6820.1972.tb04782.x

[31] James MJ, Gibson RA, Cleland LG. Dietary polyunsaturated fatty acids and inflammatory mediator production. The American Journal of Clinical Nutrition. 2000;**71** (Suppl 1):343S-348S. DOI: 10.1093/ajcn/71.1.343s

[32] Oh DY, Talukdar S, Bae EJ, Imamura T, Morinaga H, Fan W, et al. GPR120 is an omega-3 fatty acid receptor mediating potent anti-inflammatory and insulin-sensitizing effects. Cell. 2010;**142**:687-698. DOI: 10.1016/j.cell.2010.07.041

[33] Takada A, Shimizu F, Ishii Y, Ogawa M, Takao T, Koba S, et al. Plasma fatty acid composition in men over 50 in the USA and Japan. Food and Nutrition Sciences. 2018;**9**:703-710. DOI: 10.4236/fns.2018.96054

[34] Shimizu F, Ishii Y, Ogawa M, Takao T, Koba S, Takada A. Effects of various foods intakes on plasma levels of trans fatty acids in japanese old men. Food and Nutrition Sciences. 2018;**9**:797-805. DOI: 10.4236/fns.2018.97059

[35] Carnethon MR, De Chavez PJ, Zee PC, et al. Disparities in sleep characteristics by race/ethnicity in a population-based sample: Chicago Area Sleep Study. Sleep Medicine. 2016;**18**:50-55. DOI: 10.1093/ajh/hpw093

[36] Allaire J, Harris WS, Vors C, Charest A, Marin J, Jackson KH, et al. Supplementation with high-dose docosahexaenoic acid increases the Omega-3 Index more than high-dose eicosapentaenoic acid. Prostaglandins, Leukotrienes, and Essential Fatty Acids. 2017;**120**:8-14. DOI: 10.1016/j.plefa.2017.03.008

[37] Hussein N, Ah-Sing E, Wilkinson P, Leach C, Griffin BA, Millward DJ. Long-chain conversion of [13C]linoleic acid and alpha-linolenic acid in response to marked changes in their dietary intake in men. Journal of Lipid Research. 2005;**46**:269-280. DOI: 10.1194/jlr.M400225-JLR200

[38] Iso H, Kobayashi M, Ishihara J, Sasaki S, Okada K, Kita Y, et al. Intake of fish and n3 fatty acids and risk of coronary heart disease among Japanese: The Japan Public Health Center-Based (JPHC) Study Cohort I. Circulation. 2006;**113**:195-202. DOI: 10.1161/CIRCULATIONAHA.105.581355

[39] Sekikawa A, Miura K, Lee S, et al. Long chain n-3 polyunsaturated fatty acids and incidence rate of coronary artery calcification in Japanese men in Japan and white men in the USA: Population based prospective cohort study. Heart. 2014;**100**:569-573. DOI: 10.1136/heartjnl-2013-304421

[40] Sekikawa A, Horiuchi BY, Edmundowicz D, et al. A "natural experiment" in cardiovascular epidemiology in the early 21st century. Heart. 2003;**89**:255-257. DOI: 10.1136/heart.89.3.255

[41] Aung T, Halsey J, Kromhout D, et al. Associations of omega-3 fatty acid supplement use with cardiovascular disease risks: Meta-analysis of 10 trials involving 77917 individuals. JAMA Cardiology. 2018;**3**:225-234. DOI: 10.1001/jamacardio.2017.5205

[42] Marchioli R, Levantesi G. n-3 PUFAs in cardiovascular disease. International Journal of Cardiology. 2013;**170**:S33-S38. DOI: 10.1016/j.ijcard.2013.06.042

[43] Bowen KJ, Harris WS, Kris-Etherton PM. Omega-3 fatty acids and cardiovascular disease: Are there benefits? Current Treatment Options in Cardiovascular Medicine. 2016;**18**:69. DOI: 10.1007/s11936-016-0487-1

[44] Wu JH, Mozaffarian D. omega-3 fatty acids, atherosclerosis progression and cardiovascular outcomes in recent trials: New pieces in a complex puzzle. Heart. 2014;**100**:530-533. DOI: 10.1136/heartjnl-2013-305257

[45] Alexander DD, Miller PE, Van Elswyk ME, Kuratko CN, Bylsma LC. A meta-analysis of randomized controlled trials and prospective cohort studies of eicosapentaenoic and docosahexaenoic long-chain omega-3 fatty acids and coronary heart disease risk. Mayo Clinic Proceedings. 2017;**92**:15-29. DOI: 10.1016/j.mayocp.2016.10.018

[46] Maki KC, Palacios OM, Bell M, Toth PP. Use of supplemental long-chain omega-3 fatty acids and risk for cardiac death: An updated meta-analysis and review of research gaps. Journal of Clinical Lipidology. 2017;**147**:1267-1274. DOI: 10.3945/jn.117.248641. Epub 2017 May 17

[47] Del Gobbo LC,Imamura F, Aslibekyan S, et al. Omega-3 polyunsaturated fatty acid biomarkers and coronary heart disease: Pooling project of 19 cohort studies. JAMA Internal Medicine. 2016;**176**:1155-1166. DOI: 10.1001/jamainternmed.2016.2925

[48] Harris WS, Del Gobbo L, Tintle NL. The omega-3 index and relative risk for coronary heart disease mortality: Estimation from 10 cohort studies. Atherosclerosis. 2017;**262**:51-54. DOI: 10.1016/j.atherosclerosis.2017.05.007

[49] Kleber ME, Delgado GE, Lorkowski S, et al. Trans-fatty acids and mortality in patients referred for coronary angiography: The Ludwigshafen Risk and Cardiovascular Health Study. European Heart Journal. 2016;**37**:1072-1078. DOI: 10.1016/j.atherosclerosis.2017.05.007

[50] Wang Q, Afshin A, Yakoob MY, et al. Impact of nonoptimal intakes of saturated, polyunsaturated, and trans fat on global burdens of coronary heart disease. Journal of the American Heart Association. 2016;**5**(1). pii: e002891. DOI: 10.1161/JAHA.115.002891

[51] Arab L. Biomarkers of fat and fatty acid intake. Journal of Nutrition. 2003;**133**(Suppl 3):925S-932S. DOI: 10.1093/jn/133.3.925S

[52] Mori K, Ishida T, Yasuda T, et al. Serum trans-fatty acid concentration is elevated in young patients with coronary artery disease in Japan. Circulation Journal: Official Journal of the Japanese Circulation Society. 2015;**79**:2017-2025. DOI: 10.1253/circj.CJ-14-0750

[53] Valles-Colomer M, Falony G, Darzi Y, Tigchelaar EF, Wang J, Tito RY, et al. The neuroactive potential of the human gut microbiota in quality of life and depression. Nature Microbiology. 2019;**4**:623-632. DOI: 10.1038/s41564-018-0337-x